AN EXPERIMENTAL STUDY OF PITUITARY TUMOURS

GENESIS, CYTOLOGY AND HORMONE CONTENT

BY

KWA HONG GIOK

WITH 17 FIGURES

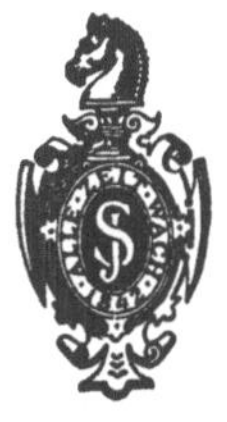

SPRINGER-VERLAG
BERLIN · GÖTTINGEN · HEIDELBERG
1961

ISBN 978-3-540-02714-0 ISBN 978-3-642-85566-5 (eBook)
DOI 10.1007/978-3-642-85566-5

Contents

I. Introduction

> ,,Let the states of equilibrium and harmony exist in perfection and a happy order will prevail through heaven and earth and all things will be nourrished and flourish.'' (MENCIUS, in ,,The Doctrine of the Mean''.)

In their natural environment the various plants and animals that have inhabited a region for ages have found a natural balance. The population of plants and animals of such a region appears to regulate itself automatically; the number of each species is kept within rather strict limits by a natural balance of forces. The introduction of a new element in such an equilibrated situation may result in a ,,disaster'' when the balance of forces that acted as a perfect self-steering device up till the introduction of that new element, fails to keep the number of that element under control. A well known example for this type of (man's) ,,interference with nature's balance of forces'' is the importation of rabbits in Australia. Because Australia's fauna did not include any of the rabbit's ,,natural enemies'' a "rabbit population explosion'' followed this unhappy decision. An equilibrated situation can become disturbed in a different way. An example of another type of (man's) "interference with nature's balance of forces'' is the introduction of modern technology and medicine in up till recently ,,backward'' countries. The ensuing raise in available food and the better hygienic standards removed the older checks on population increase such as famine and peri-natal death. This is causing a ,,human population explosion'', the extent of which can still hardly be evaluated.

When one now turns to the multi-cellular organisms it may be surmised that here also a "balance of forces'' is operating at the cellular level. Multi-cellular organisms are communities of variously differentiated cells (they are seldom if ever a mere assemblage of self-sufficient units) and they are organized so that the function of each cell depends on its relation to the whole. The number of each of the variously differentiated types of cells are in some way constantly being adjusted to the needs of the organism during growth, during tissue-repair and throughout life. A ,,balance of forces'', probably a subtle interplay of restraining and stimulating influences that act on the growth potential of each cell and that originate from neighbouring or more distant cells, is responsible.

Sometimes, however, this "balance of forces'' fails and "disaster'' results; neoplasms occur in most vertebrates and insects as well as in plants and will probably be found eventually in all multi-cellular organisms. Since neoplasms may be defined as uncontrolled new-growth of tissue, they are so to say "population explosions'' of a certain type (or of certain types) of cells. Up till recently the main trend has been to regard such "population explosions" as being caused by the ,,introduction of a new element into an equilibrated situation". When in this way the occurrence in the body of an "altered cell" (on which the normal restraining forces of the organism are not competent to act and which therefore results in cancerous growth) is compared to the introduction of the rabbit in Australia, the discovery of chemical and physical agents capable of producing mutation may be viewed to having revealed some of the mechanisms of the ,,magician's trick to produce a rabbit where none apparently existed before". It is not surprising that the possibility of a failure of the regulatory influences to be primarily at fault was disfavoured. To quote KAPLAN (1959, a): "The theory that cancer results from a disturbance of the body's normal regulatory mechanisms, originally put forth by BOVARI, seemed highly improbable when a number of specific chemical and physical carcinogenic agents, such as the hydrocarbons, the azo dyes, ultraviolet and ionising radiations were discovered."

Whether an alteration in the genes of normal somatic cells was responsible, or whether cells are constitutionally altered in some as yet unknown manner (but so that specific cytological characteristics are transmissible independently of the gene mechanism) is not relevant to the fact that the "altered cell" was considered to be primarily at fault.

Recently attention has been drawn to a number of lines of experiments emphasizing the possibility that a failure of the restraining forces of the organism may be the primary cause (KAPLAN, 1959 a and b; SMITHERS, 1959). The latter in his review expects that advances in cellular biology will provide the answers to much better questions than what (chemical) turns a normal cell into a cancer cell and mentions such questions as "What are the factors which in complex organisms transcend the cell, to unify and control a mass of protoplasm into orderly development and maintenance of a whole ? What intra-cellular mechanisms of synthesis are chiefly concerned with growth and differentiation ?"

From the view that "the interplay throughout is between cell potential and environmental restraint", the following concept of neoplastic growth is formulated by SMITHERS: "The process is seen in terms of cells with varying potentials for regeneration, normally controlled within an organismic pattern from which they may be released either by isolation from that control or by repeated demands for function which raise their growth capacity above that of the controls being exercised."

The pituitary gland seems particularly suited to study experimentally neoplastic transformation along these lines. Hormones and the nervous system are known to play a significant role in tissue organization as well as to have a trophic influence on these tissues. In the case of pituitary tissue hormone excess has been proved to cause tumour formation (oestrogens). Hormone deficiency also appears to be causative of neoplastic growth in this organ, as has been proved in mice when the deficiency concerns hormones of the thyroid gland. The anatomical integrity of the hypothalamo-pituitary system, especially its portal vessels, have been shown to be essential for the regulation of various specialized hormonal functions of the pituitary gland. This is also reflected in the cytological differentiation of the pituitary cells. The recent finding that normal pituitaries isografted subcutaneously may develop into chromophobic pituitary tumours at the site of implantation suggests that isolation from the control normally excerted by the central nervous system (hypothalamus) may result in unrestricted proliferation of (one type of) pituitary cells.

The very concept that a disturbance of the body's normal regulatory mechanism may be primarily at fault emphasizes the imperceptibility of the change from normal via hyperplasia into neoplasia and stresses that the well known difficulty of demarcating when to speak of cancerous growth during this gradual transformation is only depending on the definition used for neoplastic growth. At both ends of the scale that runs from normal via hyperplasia and benign neoplasia to malignant new growth all people will agree as to which to call cancer and which to call normal. It is in the ,,borderland'' between these extremes that difficulties arise. This applies also to pituitary tumours. Therefore a decision as to whether the induced unrestrained proliferation of cells observed is of a neoplastic nature (and if so at what stage hyperplasia has changed into neoplasia) has been evaded in the present experiments. When the various specialities studying the phenomenon of carcinogenesis have not yet settled on generally applicable and accepted definitions any verdict will be based on one's personal conviction as to which of the characteristics of cancerous growth are considered to be crucial.

The pertinent literature to pituitary tumours in mice and rats is dealt with in the following chapter. In the third chapter the pituitary tumour incidence after oestrone treatment as well as after ,,radiothyroidectomy'' in mice and rats and the growth rate of these tumours in various highly inbred strains[1] and F_1-hybrids in mice are compared. Then follows an evaluation of the Mallory tri-chrome stain in distinguishing the two types of pituitary tumours and the results obtained with a modified PAS-technique are correlated with the results of Thyroid Stimulating Hormone (TSH)-assays, which are reported in the fifth chapter. In this last chapter also some difficulties in the assay technique are mentioned, their possible significance in relation to the pathophysiology of pituitary tumors are discussed.

II. Pituitary tumours in mice and rats

A. A survey of the literature

Although the work on experimentally induced pituitary tumours covers only a period of less than two and half decades the literature has become very extensive as reflected in the many reviews covering the subject. (HORNING, 1952; GARDNER, PFEIFFER, TRENTIN and WOLSTENHOLME, 1953; FURTH, 1955; GORBMAN, 1956; FURTH, and CLIFTON, 1958;

[1] The nomenclature for highly inbred strains of mice and for their F_1-hybrids as recommended by the Committee on standardized Nomenclature for inbred Strains of Mice [Cancer Res. **12,** 602 (1952)] is followed.

FURTH, BUFFET and HARAN-GHERA, 1960; CLIFTON, 1959, etc.). Therefore it has not been the aim to give a complete review of the literature, but rather to give a comprehensive account of the background of the present work.

1. The incidence of spontaneous pituitary tumours

To evaluate the occurrence of pituitary tumours during different experimental conditions in laboratory animals, the spontaneous incidence of pituitary tumours under „normal" laboratory regimen in the species used should be taken into consideration.

a) In mice. In an extensive investigation of the incidence of spontaneous tumours in mice of the Slye-stock, covering 11,188 autopsies, SLYE, HOLMES and WELLS (1931) found only one adenoma of the pituitary.

An investigation covering four hundred pituitaries of mice of three highly inbred strains and their F_1-hybrid combinations by MÜHLBOCK (1951) revealed a fairly high incidence of spontaneously occurring pituitary adenomata in $(O_{20} \times DBA_f)F_1$ old females. The incidence in this particular F_1-hybrid is stated in a subsequent paper to be approximately 10% (MÜHLBOCK, 1953).

An incidence of approximately 8% in the old female mice of another F_1-hybrid combination $(C_{57}L \times A)F_1$ was reported by UPTON and FURTH (1955). A tendency to develop spontaneous pituitary tumours was also found in one the parent strains namely in the $C_{57}L$, whereas they did not occur in the other parent strain (A), FURTH, BUFFET and GADSDEN (1957).

In view of the extensive use of many highly inbred strains of mice in cancer research these relatively few reports on spontaneously occurring pituitary tumours in mice appear to indicate that certain unknown genetic components may favour the occurrence of this type of tumour in old mice.

The apparently sex-limited occurrence indicates that hormonal factors probably are also involved in the development of spontaneous pituitary tumours in mice and MÜHLBOCK (1953) suggested that a disruption of the subtle interplay between gonads and the pituitary may have been responsible for the tumours in old female $(O_{20} \times DBA_f)F_1$ mice. Such a hormonal imbalance between gonads and pituitary may occur incidentally or as a consequence of an inherited "abnormal" hormonal pattern. The first possibility may be illustrated by the finding of a spontaneous pituitary tumour coincident with bilateral spontaneous granulosacell tumours and multiple mammary adenocarcinoma in a mouse of the E I-strain (GARDNER, SMITH and STRONG, 1936), whereas the second possibility is illustrated by the findings in the NZY-strain of mice reported by BIELSCHOWSKY, BIELSCHOWSKY and LINDSAY (1956). In this particular strain the intact female mice showed a tendency to enlargement of the pituitary: 85% of the virgins and 93% of the breeders had pituitaries of more than 3 mg, whereas all the male and all the spayed female mice had pituitaries of less than 3 mg. In the intact females the difference between the virgins and the breeders is more strinkingly illustrated by the size of the pituitaries; none of the virgin mice had pituitaries of more than 10 mg, whereas 37% of the female breeders had pituitaries of more than 10 mg.

b) In rats. While apparently in mice the occurrence of spontaneous pituitary adenomata can be considered to be rather exceptional and limited to females, the position seems to be entirely different in rats.

Although CURTISS, BULLOCK and DUNNING (1936) did not mention a single pituitary tumour in a paper based on the study of several thousands of rats, in which spontaneous tumours in practically every other organ had been found, other authors report a fairly high incidence in a great number of strains in this species.

BRYAN, KLINCK and WOLFE (1938) found either pituitary adenomata or foci of anterior lobe cells considered to exhibit early adenomatous changes in approximately 10% of the females of the Albany strain. In a subsequent paper WOLFE, BRYAN and WRIGHT (1938) report having found a high incidence in two other strains (Vanderbilt strain: males 11.8% and females 29%; Wistar strain females 68.2% males of this strain were not studied). SAXTON (1941) and SAXTON and GRAHAM (1944) found pituitary adenomata with increasing incidence at older ages (Yale strain older than 600 days: males 60% and females 30%; in two other strains only males were studied: Sherman strain 3.6% and Wistar strain 11.1%).

2. Induced pituitary tumours

During the last two and a half decades various experimental procedures have been found to be effective in inducing pituitary tumours in mice and rats. Most of these procedures either directly or indirectly derange the homoiostatic system that regulate the hormonal "milieu interne" and such experiments emphasize the importance of a ,,hormonal imbalance" in the genesis of pituitary tumours.

a) In mice. Two types of procedure, which derange the ,,hormonal balance" between gonads and pituitary and induce pituitary tumours in this species are long term oestrogen administration and castration at an early age.

CRAMER and HORNING (1936a) were the first to report the finding of pituitary tumours in two different strains of mice, after a twice weekly application on the skin of a 0.01% oestrone solution in chloroform. Out of 12 mice autopsied after six months of treatment only 1 had a normal pituitary. Most of the literature on oestrogen-induced pituitary tumours has been reviewed by HORNING (1952) and by GARDNER, PFEIFFER, TRENTIN and WOLSTENHOLME (1953).

The importance of the genetic constitution is indicated by the reported strain difference in susceptibility to pituitary tumour induction by oestrogens: The C_{57}Bl strain showed the highest incidence, while the CBA strain appeared to be very resistant.

The liability to developing oestrogen-induced pituitary adenoma appeared to be genetically determined (GARDNER, 1941). MÜHLBOCK's observations (1951 and 1953) on continuous oestrone treatment in several strains of mice and their F_1-hybrids confirm that a genetic factor is involved.

Castration at an early age, reported by DICKIE and WOOLLEY (1949), may result in pituitary tumour formation depending on the strain of mice. A *high* incidence of pituitary tumours as a result of this experimental procedure appears to be restricted to the F_1-hybrids of the CE (and the genetically closely related DE strain) with other strains (DICKIE and LANE, 1956). Histological changes in the adrenal cortex always seemed to precede tumour development in the pituitary.

Procedures deranging the hormonal balance between the thyroid and the pituitary also appear to be effective in producing tumourous enlargement of the pituitary in mice.

GORBMAN (1949) reported the induction of pituitary tumours in mice after the administration of a thyroid-lethal dose of ^{131}I this observation was soon confirmed by others (GOLDBERG and CHAIKOFF, 1951; FURTH and BURNETT, 1951; SILBERBERG and SILBERBERG, 1954). In all strains used the incidence was reported to be extremely high (up to 95%).

Four years later MOORE, BRACKNEY and BOCK (1953) reported the finding of pituitary adenomata after prolonged treatment with thiouracil, a thyroid-blocking agent. As long term experiments with thiouracil had been carried out before in mice in many laboratories (GORBMAN, 1947; DALTON, MORRIS and DUBNIK, 1949, etc.) to study the effects of the drug on the thyroid and no changes in the pituitary suggestive of tumour formation had been reported, the positive finding of MOORE, et al. may be due to strain differences in the reaction by pituitary tumour formation to this type of treatment.

Surgical thyroidectomy also proved to be effective in C_{57}Bl mice (DENT, GADSDEN and FURTH, 1955 and 1956).

Ionizing radiations have been proved effective in causing pituitary tumours. FURTH, GADSDEN and UPTON (1953) reported on the induction of ACTH-secreting pituitary tumours in $(C_{57}L \times A)F_1$ mice, which had been exposed to intensive ionizing radiations caused by atomic detonation. Two other types of pituitary tumours — one „somato-thyrotropic" and the other „mammotropic" — were reported to have developed in mice of the same series (FURTH, 1955).

It appears that the action of ionizing irradiation can be either a direct one on the pituitary (and/or on the hypothalamic centres) or one possibly mediated by hormonal imbalances due to radiation-induced changes in the target glands, because moderate X-ray doses over the head produced pituitary tumours only in $(C_{57}L \times A)F_1$ mice, whereas whole body X-irradiation was successful in both parent strains as well as in the F_1-hybrids, (FURTH, BUFFET and GADSDEN, 1957). The negative results obtained in the C_{57}Bl strain by GORBMAN and EDELMANN (1952) emphasize that genetic factors may influence the results.

Many experimental procedures apparently can induce pituitary adenomata in mice. This is the more striking in view of the relatively low incidence of spontaneous pituitary tumours in this species.

b) In rats. The situation appears to be entirely different in rats. Whereas spontaneous pituitary tumours appear to be a not uncommon finding in this species at old age, many of the procedures that effectively induce pituitary tumours in mice have only a doubtful effect in rats. Prolonged oestrogen administration is one of the exceptions and has been proved effective in producing pituitary tumours in this species as substantiated by many reports since the findings by ZONDECK (1936) and MCEUEN, SELYE and COLLIP (1936) of pituitary adenomata in rats after oestrone administration (see reviews: HORNING, 1952; and GARDNER, PFEIFFER, TRENTIN and WOLSTENHOLME, 1953).

The pituitary tumours reported in rats bearing ovarian grafts (OBERLING, GUERIN and GUERIN, 1936; and OBERLING, SANNIE, GUERIN and GUERIN, 1939) and in the non-ovariectomized partner joined in parabiosis with an ovariectomized rat (BIELSCHOWSKY, 1954) may be interpreted to emphasize that long term hyperoestrogenization results in tumourous enlargement of the pituitary.

After bilateral castration the pituitary is reported to show microadenomas or adenomas with gonadotrophic function (HOUSSAY, HOUSSAY, CARDEZA and PINTO, 1955).

The procedures causing a hormonal imbalance on the pituitary-thyroid axis, so effective in mice, fail to provide conclusive evidence of raising the pituitary tumour incidence considerably in rats.

The technical difficulty of obtaining total ablation of the thyroid gland in rats is stressed by various authors (HOHLWEG and JUNKMANN, 1933; LEBEDEWA, 1936; GRIESBACH and PURVES, 1943), all of whom report enlargement of the pituitary gland in those rats in which the operation had been successful in removing all thyroid-tissue.

Since destruction of the thyroid by radioactive iodine has been proved such an efficient way of inducing pituitary tumours in mice, several groups of workers have tried without success to induce pituitary tumours in rats by this technically simple method of obtaining total elimination of thyroid function (EDELMANN, 1954 — see the discussion following his paper). FURTH, DENT, BURNETT and GADSDEN (1955) reported that analysis of the data in their series of „radiothyroidectomized" rats revealed that the pituitary tumour incidence in the ^{131}I treated group was not higher than in the controls.

SEIFTER, EHRICH and HUDYMA (1949) reported pituitary adenomata in rats fed thyroid-blocking agents in their diets from weaning until death. The small number of animals reaching sufficiently old age in both experimental (3 rats) and control (3 rats) groups makes it difficult to evaluate the reported tumour incidence.

CLAUSEN (1956) found that after administration of 0.2% thiouracil in drinking water for 24 months the pituitary weights were 30% over the controls. For comparison, after long term oestrogen administration the pituitary weights in the experimental groups often are more than 1000% of the values in the controls. CLAUSEN reported finding one to three nodular growths in the pituitaries in all of the ten treated rats as against one out of five control rats.

The coincidental finding of pituitary adenomata, described as basophile, and thyroid hyperplasia in old rats of two strains are considered to suggest that a chronic thyroxin deficiency produced by an I-deficient diet may have been the cause of this syndrome (BIELSCHOWSKY, 1953). AXELRAD and LEBLOND (1955) reported enlargement of the anterior pituitary in 10 out of 26 autopsied rats that had received an I-deficient diet for $9^1/_2$ months or longer.

Seven had macroscopic tumours weighing up to 258 mg. No data are available on the spontaneous pituitary tumour incidence in their stock of rats.

Ionizing irradiation appears to increase the pituitary tumour incidence in rats. VAN DYKE, SIMPSON, KONEFF and TOBIAS (1959) reported that in rats irradiated with a high energy deuteron beam the lower doses used (945 and 1575 rep) increased the incidence of pituitary tumours. Between the 16th and 24th months histological adenomata were found in 32% of the control group and in the 975 rep — and the 1575 rep groups the incidences were respectively 95% and 65% (mean 3.1 per gland against 1.6 per gland in the controls).

Diets containing p-Fluoroacetanilide, o-Hydroxyacetanilide and 2.3-Dimethylanilide have been reported to increase the pituitary tumour incidence in female rats of the Buffalo strain from 10 to 15% in the controls to 50 to 60% in the experimental groups (MORRIS, LOMBARD, WAGNER and WEISBURGER, 1957).

As the spontaneous pituitary tumour incidence under normal laboratory conditions appears to be very high in some strains of rats at old age, it is difficult to accept unreservedly the reported incidence in various experimental conditions as a consequence of the treatment (FURTH, 1955; GORBMAN, 1956). This appears to apply especially to the experiments aimed at chronic thyroxin deficiency.

3. Concepts on pituitary physiology that have contributed to current theories on pituitary tumour induction mechanisms

In the elucidation of the relationship between the pituitary and its various target glands the description of involutionary changes in the gonads (CROWE, CUSHING and HOMANS, 1910) and in the thyroid (SMITH, 1916 and 1927) after hypophysectomy was followed by a stream of anatomical and physiological research which led to the concept of a reciprocal regulatory action between the secretions of the pituitary and the thyroid, and between the pituitary and the gonads, postulated respectively by ARON, VAN CAULERT and STAHL (1931) and by MOORE and PRICE (1932). A similar reciprocal regulatory relationship appears to exist between the pituitary and the adrenal cortex (SAYERS and SAYERS, 1947).

a) The negative feed-back mechanisms. Thus information on pituitary function obtained by various methods of investigation has led to the concept of a reciprocal regulatory action between the release of the various pituitary trophic hormones and the release of the specific hormone by the respective target glands; a low blood-level of a specific target gland hormone effects a release and an increased production of the pituitary trophic principle, which stimulates the target gland involved, whilst a high blood level of the hormone of that target gland is thought to inhibit the release (and production) of the pituitary trophic principle. It has been compared to the self-steering devices developed in technology (HOSKINS, 1949), such as the automatic regulation of the room temperature by thermostats, the automatic volume control in radio receivers, etc., which are known as servo mechanisms or (negative) feed-back systems.

For the pituitary-ovarian interrelation experimental results appear to be in agreement with the servo mechanism theory: *bio assays* of pituitary gonadotrophin content indicate a sharp rise after castration (EVANS and SIMPSON, 1929, etc.) and a decrease after the administration of gonadal hormones; *parabiosis experiments* (WITSCHI, 1937) show a high gonadotrophin level after castration; the successful *tumour induction* in the ovary transplanted into the spleen (BISKIND and BISKIND, 1944) in ovariectomized female mice and rats may also be explained by the servo mechanism theory.

The same trends have been found for the interrelationship between pituitary and thyroid (ADAMS, 1946; D'ANGELO, 1954) as well as for the pituitary and the adrenal cortex.

It should be appreciated that the system as outlined above is a gross oversimplification of reality. This is emphasized by the recent findings that the integrity of the hypothalamo-pituitary system appears to be essential for the functional and morphological differentiation of the pituitary gland (EVERETT, 1956).

The hypothalamic centres either form a link in the postulated feed-back systems, prolactin secretion appearing to be regulated by the degree of inhibition of the pituitary gland by the hypothalamic centres involved, whereas ACTH secretion seems to be regulated by the degree of stimulation by the centres, or else the hypothalamic centres modulate a direct effect on the pituitary of the blood level of the hormone of the target gland involved (HARRIS, 1955; ROTHBALLER, 1957; BROWN-GRANT, 1957, etc.).

Such findings imply that the application of the concept of feed-back mechanisms calls for caution when pituitary or pituitary tumour function and morphology are studied in transplantation experiments. Whereas transplantation of the target glands, (the gonads, thyroid and probably also the adrenal cortex), leaves intact the reciprocal control presumed by the feed-back concept, any experimental condition interfering with the integrity of the hypothalamo-pituitary system, (such as transplantation of the normal or tumourously enlarged pituitary or damage by pressure of a pituitary tumour of the hypothalamic centres involved), by itself may cause a disruption of the postulated reciprocal control.

b) Present tendency to assign the various functions of the pituitary to different cell types. One of the two main methods of determining the specific cellular origin of the hormones of the pituitary has been the attempt to correlate the changes in the numerical proportions of different cell types with various physiological states. The other method tries to discover directly the secretory activity of the hypophysis by an analysis of the changes in various physiological conditions in certain structural

Table 1. *Present trend to ascribe the production of each pituitary hormone to a specific cell type of the anterior pituitary*

Pituitary hormone	Staining with Mallory tri-chrome	Special methods used and/or special characteristics of the cells	Author
growth hormone (STH)	acidophiles		see review, PEARSE (1952, a)
prolactin (LTH)	acidophiles	the acidophile granule fraction obtained by differential centrifugation gave positive crop-sac reaction	HERLANT (1952)
	acidophiles	orangeophile	LACOUR, 1950
	acidophiles	carminophile	DAWSON, 1946
prolactin (LTH) and/or LH	acidophiles	carminophile staining due to sulfhydril and/or disulfide groups, therefore containing either prolactin, LH, or both	LADMAN and BARRNETT (1954) LADMAN and BARRNETT (1956)
ACTH	acidophiles	acidophile granule fraction obtained by fractionated centrifugation induced marked adrenal hypertrophy in rats	STIGLIANI, MAGGI and FANFANI, 1954
	chromophobes	"ACTH does not appear to be secreted by either acidophiles or basophiles and therefore is presumed to be secreted by the chromophobes" (in dogs)	PURVES and GRIESBACH, 1956
	basophiles	the aldehyde-fuchsin positive basophiles, inferred from their reaction to stress, etc.	KIEF (1956)
TSH	basophiles	PAS-positive cells with angular cell outlines, centrally located, staining aldehyde-fuchsin positive	PURVES and GRIESBACH (1951, a and b) HALMI, 1952, b
LH (ICSH)	basophiles	PAS-positive cells with rounded contours, centrally located, aldehyde-fuchsin negative	PURVES and GRIESBACH, 1954, 1955
		PAS-red	RENNELS, HILDEBRAND and FINERTY, 1956
FSH	basophiles	PAS-positive cells with rounded contours, peripherally located, aldehyde-fuchsin negative	PURVES et al., 1954, 1955
		PAS-purper	RENNELS et al. 1956

characteristics which the anterior lobe cells have in common with other secretory cells. The changes in the Golgi apparatus, in the mitochondria and in the nucleus and its nucleolus are thought to reflect the metabolic state of the cells whilst the specific granules are held to be the secretory products of the cell or their precursors.

By various staining methods, such as Mallory's triple stain three main cell types were generally recognized: the acidophiles, the basophiles and the chromophobes. The possible relationship between these three main cell types has given rise to many schemas, which according to SEVERINGHAUS (1937) may be divided into two groups; the first assumes that there is but one cell type in the anterior lobe and that the chromophobes, acidophiles and basophiles represent various phases of the same cell, the second assumes that acidophiles and basophiles are separate and distinct cells, independently related to the chromophobes.

Earlier evidence pointed to the chromophiles as the only two pituitary cell types, that elaborate physiologically active principles. It is not surprising that the existence of only two true pituitary hormones has been surmised. RIDDLE (1937) suggested that too many hormones had been postulated, he preferred to call the different products which had been obtained „hormone fragments"; the two "true hormones" being: one with lactogenic, adrenotrophic and growth effects secreted by the acidophiles and the other with gonadotrophic and possibly thyrotrophic effects secreted by the basophiles. COLLIP (1939) also visualized two large hormone molecules with prosthetic groups responsible for the reported physiologic activities, which are "chemically dissected" in the various purification procedures.

Since 1935 the chromophiles have been further differentiated morphologically by the use of modified staining methods (COWIE and FOLLEY, 1955). Table 1 is compiled randomly from current literature and reflects the present trend to distinguish as many hormone producing pituitary cell types as there appear to be pituitary hormones. The allocation of ACTH production appears to be still in dispute. This may be compared to the situation for the production site of TSH up till 1946 (ADAMS, 1946) when the votes appeared to be equally divided among the basophile and the acidophile cells. The problem of the allocation of the production of the various pituitary hormones to specific and distinct cell types has not been settled and becomes even more complicated by the apparently existing species differences (PURVES and GRIESBACH, 1957b). A universally accepted opinion has not yet been reached. Even the question whether each of them is produced in a separate and distinct cell type seems to be still unsettled.

4. Present concepts on pituitary tumour induction mechanisms

Hormones are organic compounds secreted by certain specific body cells and, although reaching all tissues, they appear to affect only those that are competent to respond to their particular stimulus. They regulate the organism's demand for functional activity of their target tissue and may be divided into "general metabolic" (thyroxine, insulin, growth hormone, etc.) and "organotrophic" hormones (oestrone, etc. gonadotrophins etc.) according to the distribution of their target tissue which may be either scattered more or less throughout the organism or restricted mainly to one or more organs.

Some of the hormones not only regulate the function of their target tissue, but affect also the "population dynamics" of their target tissue cells, thus such hormones have a stimulatory action on the function of their target organs as well as a trophic effect on them.

Shifts in hormonal balance, either occurring incidentally or experimentally induced, may lead to a prolonged hormonal hyperstimulation and in various hormone sensitive tissues cancerous growth may ensue because of such a long sustained super-normal action of the particular hormone for which the tissue is a target. Only those hormones, which have a trophic effect in addition to their stimulatory action on the function of their targetorgans appear to be carcinogenic in this sence (MÜHLBOCK, 1959).

It has already been mentioned above, that derangements of hormonal balance are thought to be responsible for the spontaneous, and most of the experimental pituitary tumours in mice and rats, it can be expected therefore that some parallels can be drawn between the processes of carcinomatous transformation in the different target organs and in the pituitary respectively.

Carcinomatous transformation in the target glands is a gradual process and appears to begin with physiological response of hypertrophy as a consequence of stimulation and proceeds via adenoma formation to cancerous growth. It is extremely difficult to define when it should be called cancer and this will depend largely on what criterion is held to be conclusive. The same considerations apply to pituitary tumour formation.

As to the causative factor in the induction of tumours a parallel may also be drawn between hormone-induced tumours in other organs and the oestrogen-induced pituitary tumour. If the pituitary is defined as one of the target-tissues for oestrogens and if oestrogens exert a stimulative action on pituitary function as well as a trophic effect on the pituitary gland, the pituitary tumour induction by long sustained excessive oestrogen levels falls into the general concept of tumour induction by hormonal derangement.

The other types of hormonal derangement leading to tumourous enlargement of the pituitary, however, are not covered by this general concept of tumour induction by a supernormal action of hormones because an excess of hormone acting on the pituitary is not involved. The recognition that the reciprocal control of pituitary hormone secretion and the secretion of hormones by several of its target glands is maintained according to the principles of a negative feed-back system, makes it plausible that, besides a chronic excess of a hormone like oestrone, a deficiency of some of the other target gland hormones may lead to induction of tumourous growth in the pituitary.

The observation that only those hormones that have a trophic effect besides their stimulatory action on function, are carcinogenic has its counterpart in the observed fact that a chronic deficiency of some hormones can induce tumourous enlargement of the pituitary, whereas a chronic deficiency of others apparently fail to do so. For example a chronic deficiency of gonadal hormones following castration results in an enhanced gonadotrophin output by the pituitary but, usually, fails to induce tumourous enlargement of the pituitary, whereas a chronic thyroid hormone deficiency almost always induces pituitary tumours in mice besides inducing an enhanced TSH secretion. The disruption of the negative feedback relationship is also probably responsible for the trophic action on the pituitary gland. This can be visualized as being effected by a decrease, or the complete abolition, of the inhibition of the mitotic activity in the pituitary normally excerted by the appropriate target gland hormone.

Thus for the pituitary gland the mechanism of induction of tumourous enlargement may be assumed to be the result of either stimulation of the mitotic activity in the pituitary by an excess of a hormone (oestrogen), or abolition of the inhibition of the mitotic activity in the pituitary by a hormone deficiency (negative feed back).

Depending on one's view of the relationship between the morphologically different cells in the normal pituitary, as to whether they are various functional and morphological phases of the same cell, or functionally and morphologically separate and distinct cell types, independently related to the pituitary "mother"-cell, different concepts of the origin and nature of pituitary tumours are possible.

a) Each specific pituitary cell type, producing its own hormone, may give rise to a monomorphous, monohormonal pituitary tumor. The present trend to ascribe the production of each of the different known pituitary hormones to a specific cell type in the anterior lobe of the hypophysis has been discussed above and forms the basis of FURTH's ideas on pituitary tumours as he conceives the pituitary to be "a mosaic of different functional cell types independently regulating specific functions" (FURTH, BUFFET and HARAN-GHERA, 1960), each of these cell types regulating (the hormone production, the growth etc. of) their target glands and in their turn being regulated by stimuli from these target glands. The disruption of one of these servo controls may be followed by a hyperfunction and a hypertrophy of the pituitary cell type involved. This hypertrophy, first ad magnitudinem and later ad numerum, may lead to tumourous enlargement of the pituitary. On this basis six different types of pituitary tumours may be expected to occur.

The schematical representation in Table 2 of the pituitary tumours that have been induced in mice under various experimental conditions, has been based on the concept that these tumours represent different "monomorphous, monohormonal masses" and should therefore be a fair approximation to FURTH's view on this subject as he stated: "The observations thus far made favour the view that by design and serendipity it will be possible to break up the pituitary gland into as many hormone secreting units as it posesses. The available facts are meager, but they point to the existence of different celltypes, some of which secrete only one trophic hormone" (FURTH, 1955).

FURTH et al. (FURTH, DENT, BURNETT and GADSDEN, 1955; DENT, GADSDEN and FURTH, 1955) ascribe a major role, if not the only causative one to the chronic thyroid hormone(s) deficiency induced by eliminating the thyroid gland by a thyroid-lethal dose of radioactive iodine in the pituitary tumour induction mechanism in mice.

Table 2. *Schematical classification of pituitary tumours in mice and rats*

Proliferating cell type		Hormone (presumed to be) produced	Experimental condition	Type of pituitary stimulation
theoretical	reported			
beta-basophile	degranulated beta-basophile; chromophobe	TSH (thyrotrophin, etc.)	surgical thyroidectomy, „radiothyroidectomy", thyroid-blocking agents, I-deficient diet	disruption of servo mechanism between thyroid gland and pituitary, due to chronic thyroid hormone(s) deficiency
acidophile, „prolactin-producing type"	degranulated acidophile; chromophobe (basophile)	prolactin. (luteotrophin, mammotrophic hormone, lactogenic hormone, etc.)	continuous oestrogen treatment, hyperoestrogenization mediated by dysfunction of gonads and/or adrenals, spontaneous, radiation induced[1], or following early castration[2]	oestrogens acting as specific stimulators of prolactin producing cells
acidophile, „ACTH-producing type"	„predominantly chromophobic, small number of cells contained coarse acidophilic granules"	ACTH (adrenocorticotrophin, etc.)	radiation induced[1]	radiation induced damage to the adrenals: disruption of the servo mechanism between adrenals and pituitary
acidophile „growth hormone producing type"	small chromophobes	growth hormone. (STH, somatotrophin, etc.)	radiation induced[1]	unknown
delta-basophile, „FSH-producing type"	basophile	FSH	early castration[2]	disruption of the servo mechanism between gonads and pituitary
delta-basophile, „LH-producing type"	basophile	LH (ICSH, etc.)	early castration[2]	disruption of the servo mechanism between gonads and pituitary

[1] Three types of pituitary tumours were reported to occur in the series of mice exposed to ionizing radiations.

[2] Position of the pituitary tumours reported after early castration in the schematical classification is uncertain (see text).

On the basis of the negative feed-back principle it may be expected that the thyroid hormone(s) deficiency will result in a hyperfunction of the TSH-producing cells and that ultimately these cells will give rise to tumour formation. The opinion of HALMI and GUDE (1954) that such tumours are derived from "degranulated" beta-basophiles, presumed to be comparable to the thyrotrophin-producing-basophiles described by PURVES and GRIESBACH (1951), HALMI (1952), etc. in the rat, fits well into this concept.

As it is irreleveant how the deficiency of the thyroid hormone(s) is achieved, the pituitary enlargement and adenoma formation after surgical thyroidectomy, long term treatment with thyroid-blocking agents and an I-deficient diet should be classified under the same heading.

The mechanism of oestrogen administration resulting in pituitary adenomata cannot be explained by a disruption of a simple model servo mechanism. GARDNER (1948) postulated cellular changes in the pituitary caused by a continuous suppression of the secretion of one or more of the pituitary hormones and leading to tumourous enlargement and he suggested (1953) that oestrogens induce tumorigenic senility changes in the pituitary. MÜHLBOCK (1953) suggested that disruption of the subtle interplay between gonads and pituitary is responsible for the spontaneously occurring as well as for the oestrone-induced pituitary tumours in mice and draws attention to the similarity structurally as well as functionally between the oestrone-induced and the spontaneous pituitary tumours in this species. The striking similarity between the oestrone-induced and the spontaneously occurring pituitary tumours in rats had been stressed by WOLFE, BRYAN and WRIGHT (1938).

A theory which brings the oestrogen-induced pituitary tumours in line with the concept of "monomorphous, monohormonal masses" i.e. different types of pituitary tumours, each consisting of secreting pituitary cells of one type only, is the following proposed by CLIFTON and MEYER (1956b): oestrogen acts as a specific stimulator of the acidophiles and pre-acidophilic chromophobes (reserve cells), which secrete prolactin: It induces cellular hypertrophy (cell volume increase, hypertrophy "ad magnitudinem") and enhances mitotic activity. When oestrogen is made to act continuously the increase of cell volume and the intense vascularization are held responsible for the enlargement of the pituitary in the first phase; the continuously heightened mitotic activity exceeds the requirements of normal cell replacement and an increase in numbers of the cell type involved (hypertrophy "ad numerum") will take place. This process does not lead to an appreciable enlargement of the gland in the initial period, but as this cell increase proceeds according to a geometrical progression, once a certain point has been reached enlargement of the pituitary will become very rapid. The oestrogen-induced pituitary tumours therefore are considered to be derived from the prolactin secreting cells.

The spontaneous pituitary tumours, the pituitary tumours occurring after gonadectomy and the prolactin secreting type of pituitary tumour induced by ionizing radiations have been classified under the same heading as the oestrogen-induced pituitary tumours in the schematical representation, based on the assumption that the common hormonal disturbance causing all these types of pituitary tumours is hyperoestrogenization.

The morphological description of spontaneous pituitary tumours in mice (MÜHLBOCK, 1953; FURTH and CLIFTON, 1958) and rats (WOLFE, BRYAN and WRIGHT, 1938) and of the prolactin secreting type of pituitary tumour arising in mice after irradiation (FURTH, 1955; FURTH and CLIFTON, 1958) agree with the proposed position in the schematical classification. The tumours are described as containing mainly chromophobic cells, a few cells still containing coarse acidophilic granules. The descriptions are suggestive of "fully degranulated and degranulating acidophile cells".

The position of the pituitary tumours arising after early castration, however, is uncertain. The sequence of events: gonadectomy — occurrence of adrenal changes, which are associated with signs of hyperoestrogenization — pituitary tumours — and mammary hyperplasia, is open to different interpretations after the stage of hyperoestrogenization has been established:

The tumourous enlargement of the pituitary can be interpreted as the usual sequel to hyperoestrogenization caused in this case by the adrenal new growth and not directly related to the ablation of the gonads. The reported mammary hyperplasia is consistent with the enhanced prolactin output that may be expected of oestrogen-induced pituitary tumours. The disappearance of the typical "castration cells" in the pituitary of castrated rats prior to the adenomatous enlargement of the pituitary would suggest, that the effect of castration on the pituitary has been effectively counteracted by the oestrogens from the adrenal new growths.

The morphological description of the pituitary adenomas and tumours as basophilic by two independent groups of investigators employing different species indicate, however, that these tumours are considered to consist of FSH and/or LH secreting cells rather than of acidophilic prolactin secreting cells (DICKIE and WOOLLEY, 1949, etc; HOUSSAY, HOUSSAY, CARDEZA and PINTO, 1955). Moreover in the rat it was proved by parabiosis experiments that such pituitaries secreted very high amounts of gonadotrophins.

FURTH (1955) mentioned both possibilities, but appears to regard these tumours as prolactin producing as later it is stated: "Attempts to induce gonadotrophic tumours have thus far been unsuccessful . . ." (FURTH and CLIFTON, 1958).

After exposure to ionizing irradiation several types of pituitary tumours seem to appear. The hormonal function of the pituitary tumours appears to have been analysed only arising in mice and in the same series of mice three functionally differents types have been found, viz: an ACTH-, a prolactin- and a growth hormone -secreting type.

The prolactin producing type has been mentioned above and classified under the oestrogen-induced pituitary tumours. The observation, that ovariectomy prevented the development of this type of tumour (FURTH and CLIFTON, 1958) emphasize that ovarian dysfunction following irradiation may be involved.

For the mechanism of induction of the ACTH secreting type FURTH (1955) proposed as a working hypothesis that "the inciting cause is damage to the adrenal, with sustained depression of this organ".

A hypothesis for the induction mechanism of the growth hormone producing type apparently could not be given, for FURTH and CLIFTON (1958) stated: "We have no idea what regulates somatotropes (cells producing growth hormone) and thus how to cheat their feed-back mechanism and make them become tumourous".

Therefore a constant relationship between a well established type of hormonal imbalance and a definite functional type of a pituitary tumour seems to be restricted, if the controversial pituitary tumour arising after early castration is excluded, to two types, namely between hyper-oestrogenization and prolactin producing pituitary tumour, and between thyroid hormone(s) deficiency and TSH producing pituitary tumour. The causal relationship in the latter case was suggested, when the administration of thyroxin (GOLDBERG and CHAIKOFF, 1951) and implantation of thyroid tissue (GORBMAN, 1952) was shown to prevent the development of pituitary tumours after the complete destruction of the thyroid gland by ^{131}I.

In fact the theory that the actual development of a pituitary tumour can be induced by stimuli from the target organ via the negative feed-back mechanism is based solely on the evidence that thyroid hormone(s) deficiency is effective in this way. As the concept of a monomorphous, monohormonal pituitary tumour necessarily must be based on the assumption that only one functional cell type of the pituitary is stimulated to hyperfunction and consequently to proliferation by the experimental procedure, consideration should be given to the working hypothesis formulated by GORBMAN (1956) according to which single stimuli, or removal of inhibitions may not induce tumourous enlargement of the pituitary although double stimuli may do so.

Contrary to FURTH et al., GORBMAN and his co-workers have always considered the ionizing radiation from radioactive iodine to be an important co-factor in pituitary tumour induction after the administration of a thyroid-destructive dose of ^{131}I. The radiation is thought to contribute either by a direct tumourigenic action on the pituitary cell, or by an indirect action invoking a "stress-like" stimulus possibly involving the adrenals, or in both ways.

This "stress-like" stimulus is suggested as a possible "common denominator" in all experimentally induced hormonal imbalances leading to pituitary tumour formation. It is thought to be brought about either by ,,toxic" side-effects in long term treatment with high doses of thiouracil compounds or in chronic hyperoestrogenization or by the trauma of surgery and the loss and re-establishment of parathyroid function in the surgical thyroidectomy experiments of DENT, GADSDEN and FURTH (1955), or by the radiation in the case of "radiothyroidectomy".

The double stimuli hypothesis has been inspired by experiments reported by EDELMANN (1954) proving the co-tumourigenic action of ionizing radiations in C_{57}Bl mice after castration and after thyroid destruction with low doses of radioactive iodine, irrespective of the source of the radiations (X-ray or radiosodium) and irrespective of the site to which the X-rays were delivered (head only, body only, or whole body). Neither of these treatments alone resulted in pituitary adenoma formation, nor did radiation alone. Castration as well as thyroid destruction followed by additional irradiation, however, resulted in tumourous enlargement of the pituitary. EDELMANN suggested that the increased demand for ACTH following irradiation in addition to the increased demand for the other trophic hormone, gonadotrophins or thyrotrophin, respectively may have tipped the balance and caused adenomatous growth of the pituitary.

This idea of a "dual secretory load" i.e. ACTH + gonadotrophins, ACTH + TSH, ACTH + prolactin, etc., is one of the possibilities GORBMAN (1956) contemplates as the mechanism by which his "common denominator, bodily stress" may contribute to the development of pituitary tumours. But if the increased demand for more than one trophic hormone is considered to cause tumourous growth of the pituitary, then more than one functional cell type of the pituitary is considered to have been stimulated to hyperfunction and consequently the proliferation of more than one cell type must have contributed to the pituitary tumour formation. Thus the resulting pituitary tumour should be understood to be a "bi-hormonal, bi-morphous pituitary tumour", or even a "multi-hormonal, multi-morphous" tumour, rather than a "monohormonal, monomorphous pituitary tumour". FURTH et. al. have more recently mentioned the possibility of "mixed tumours" too, but appear to restrict it to the pituitary tumours resulting from irradiation: "... It is possible, however, that some primary pituitary tumours contain several types of neoplastic cells, which could be separated through passages in variously conditioned hosts" (FURTH, BUFFETT and HARAN-GHERA, 1960).

If the idea of six separate and distinct pituitary cell types each producing only its own pituitary hormone is abandoned the other extreme view on the origin and nature of these functionally active pituitary tumours is reached:

b) The omnipotent pituitary amphophile cell, capable of producing every pituitary hormone, giving rise to potentially multi-hormonal, amphophile, pituitary tumours. The theoretical possibility that a pituitary cell type may produce more than one trophic hormone seems to be essential for the understanding of some pituitary tumours in man, according to RUSSFIELD, REINER and KLAUS (1956). They advanced two hypotheses: "a) amphophile cells may secrete growth hormone, ACTH, thyrotrophin, gonadotrophin, and mammotrophin, although not necessarily simultaneously, and b) target organ deficiency may be involved in the pathogenesis of some pituitary tumours ...".

The relationship visualized between the "amphophile" cell and the other pituitary cell types depends on whether the various types of cells are considered to represent: groups of separate and distinct cells or the various phases of one and the same cell.

Thus the "amphophile" cells may be conceived to be the direct descendants of the undifferentiated chromophobe „mother" cell[1] and persisting in the pituitary along with the fully differentiated and functionally specialized cell types and still potentially capable of producing every pituitary hormone.

Alternatively according to the second concept "TSH producing basophile" cells, "prolactin producing eosinophile" cells, etc. and "amphophile" cells may change one into another.

The status of the "amphophile" cell is not clear. The capacity of its granules to take either red or blue stain with the Mallory tri-chrome technique, depending on the fixation technique and P_h used, is reflected in the name and suggests that these cells are considered to be a separate group, which can not be classified either under the eosinophile or under the basophile cell types. The first of the above mentioned possibilities appears to have been adopted. Therefore it may be opportune to compare this concept with the ideas of SEVERINGHAUS (1933, 1937), who is a proponent of early and irreversible differentiation into the eosinophile and basophile cell types, since his extreme view appears to preclude the possibility of undifferentiated cells in the mature pituitary.

The morphological description of the "amphophile" cell as a sparsely granulated cell (RUSSFIELD, et al., etc.) suggests that the group or groups of pituitary cells covered by this term probably include both the "partly degranulated basophile" as well as the "partly degranulated acidophile" cells of SEVERINGHAUS. The essential difference between the two concepts is the relationship of these cells to the "basophile" and "acidophile" cell types of the pituitary.

Whereas the observation on which the amphophile cell concept is based is the variable staining properties of its granules, the essential observation in the concept of SEVERINGHAUS is the "acidophile type" and the "basophile type" of Golgi apparatus in the pituitary cells. According to SEVERINGHAUS the morphology of the Golgi apparatus is so different for the acidophile line and the basophile line of cells, that even its "negative image" in the routinely stained pituitary sections are of diagnostic value. By this criterion it is claimed to be possible to divide the chromophobes into (pre-)acidophilic and (pre-)basophilic types, and to classify the degranulating and even the fully degranulated chromophile cells as being derived from either acidophile or basophile cells.

However, Golgi apparatus typical for the acidophile or basophile lines of cells appears to be restricted to some species only. They can not be differentiated in man, mouse, etc. (PEARSE, 1952b), whereas in the rat and in some other species this appears to be possible. Although the con-

[1] In this regard the possibility put forward by HERLANT (1943, quoted by WOLFE, 1949) should be mentioned in which the pituitary chromophobe cells are thought to produce all the trophic hormones in sufficient quantities to meet the basal need. The specialized chromophile cells are thought to release their specific hormone when the organism requires more than the normal amount.

cept of „amphophile" cells may therefore not be relevant to the pituitary of the rat, the striking similarity of the morphological description of a non-granular (degranulated), enlarged cell, with a giant nucleus and the possible endocrinal significance of the "hypertrophied amphophile" and the "functionally active, hypertrophied chromophobe" cell (SEVERINGHAUS, 1937) is noteworthy. The most interesting feature of the "functionally active, hypertrophied chromophobe" cell is that the criterion of the specific types of Golgi apparatus apparently may fail for this type of cell and it is stated that it can be difficult, if not impossible, to recognize whether it has been derived from a degranulating acidophile or a basophile cell (SEVERINGHAUS, 1937). This difficulty is also endorsed by WOLFE (1949). Evidence of hypersecretion of any of the pituitary hormones by pituitary tumours composed of such "non-granular, enlarged cells with giant nuclei" seems to be explicate by either concept of cellular relationships in the pituitary; by definition in the "amphophile" cell concept and by the technical difficulties of classifying these cells according to the concept of SEVERINGHAUS.

The other property of the granules of the "amphophile" cell, i.e. their "weakly PAS-positive" reaction, might give more information about the relation of the "amphophile" cell to the other pituitary cell types. One possibility is that the "amphophile" cells include both the "thyrotrophin producing basophile" cell and the "gonadotrophin(s) producing basophile" cell(s) of PURVES and GRIESBACH (1951 a and b), the "beta-basophile" and the "delta-basophile" cells of HALMI (1952a) respectively. This interpretation of the "amphophile" cell concept would indicate a profound difference of opinion on the endocrine significance of the PAS-positive cells, and is also suggested by the use of the term "amphophile" for the tumours occurring in the pituitaries of mice after the administration of a thyroid-destructive dose of ^{131}I by BURT, LANDING and SOMMERS (1954).

BURT, et al. recognized two types of "basophiles" and in the early post-administration period the larger ones, with indistinct and often irregular cell outlines, were found to hypertrophy and increase in numbers. They stated that these cells in the mouse pituitary closely resemble the "thyrotrophic basophile" cells, which were described in the rat pituitary by PURVES and GRIESBACH (1951). Thus BURT, et al. appear to be in agreement with HALMI and GUDE (1954). However, an essential difference between HALMI and GUDE and PURVES and GRIESBACH on the one hand and BURT, et. al. on the other in the estimate of the hormonal functions of the cells is suggested, when the latter authors also mention the close resemblance of these cells to the „sparsely granulated basophile" (MELLGREN, 1945) or the "amphophile" cell.

A comparison of the descriptions[1] of the cellular changes in the pituitary of mice after destruction of their thyroid glands by radioactive iodine

[1] BURT, et al. describe that the "amphophile" cells occasionally became vacuolated as hyperplasia increased, losing most or all of their granules. The nuclei increased sometimes tremendously and showed enlarged nucleoli. These "thyroidectomy cells" are said to bear a striking resemblance to the "hypertrophied amphophile" cells in

suggests that the PAS-positive cells described as "beta-basophile" and as "delta-basophile" by HALMI and GUDE are considerd by BURT, et al. to be various phases of "amphophile" cells.

The concluding remark of BURT et al. "... that the sparsely granulated amphophilic family of cells, through the production of some types of trophic hormones, may play a more important role in the endocrine imbalance of tumour formation than has been generally recognized", also indicates that their view on the hormonal function of the "amphophile" cell is nearer to the omnipotent "amphophile" cell of RUSSFIELD, et al. (1956) than to the ideas of PURVES and GRIESBACH, who are decided proponents of the view that each differentiated cell type produces only its specific hormone.

In the first morphological descriptions the oestrone-induced (CRAMER and HORNING, 1936 a and b) as well as the radioactive iodine induced (GORBMAN, 1949) pituitary tumours in mice were designated chromophobic tumours. One of the objections against the description of these functionally active tumours as "chromophobic" appears to be the connotation of physiological inactivity, which first this term has acquired (BURT, SOMMERS and LANDING, 1954).

This semantic pitfall may have played a part in the opinion expressed by CRAMER and HORNING (1938), that the finding of signs in the endocrine glands similar to those found after destruction of the hypophysis by disease or after its surgical removal, are accounted for by the fact that the great increase in the mass of the pituitary gland consists of chromophobe, and accordingly physiologically inactive, cells. It is interesting to note that they described cells with large vesicular nuclei with distinct nucleoli. In pituitary cells (WOLFE, 1949) and in pituitary tumour cells (BURT, et al., 1954), such nuclei are considered to indicate active protein synthesis reflecting physiological activity. Thus it appears that the cells of the pituitary tumours described by CRAMER and HORNING should be considered to show enhanced physiological activity rather than inactivity. The apparent paradox of finding them in combination with atrophied target glands might as well be explained by considering the functional state of the target glands to have been the cause of the pituitary adenomata instead of having been effected by the physiologically inactive tumour. Assuming that these pituitary tumours are "amphophilic" in the

---

the human pituitary. In fact the hyperplastic cells of their mouse pituitary adenomata could be made to show the staining charateristics of either "basophile" or "acidophile" cells and could be made to show the PAS reaction either strongly positive, or weakly positive or even negative, depending on the Ph as well as on the fixation technique used.

The description of HALMI and GUDE mentions also an increase of the PAS-positive elements in the early post-radiation periods, but this increase is ascribed to an increase of the gonadotrophin producing "delta-basophile" cells. The thyrotrophin producing "beta-basophile" cells are stated to degranulate and hypertrophy and these latter cells are thought to give rise to the pituitary tumours composed of "degranulated beta-basophile" cells. The ,,delta-basophile" cells have almost disappeared by then. The occasional PAS-positive cells in such tumours are considered to be remnants of the "delta-basophile" cells.

sense of RUSSFIELD, et al., the production of more than one trophic hormone would be expected as a result of this multiple target gland insufficiency.

The reported increase of pituitary hormonal production of ACTH (MEITES and TURNER, 1948; NADEL, JOSEPHSON and MULAY, 1950), of prolactin (MEITES and TURNER, 1948; MÜHLBOCK, 1953; MEYER and CLIFTON, 1956) and of TSH (CLIFTON and MEYER, 1956 a) after oestrogen treatment apparently agrees with such a view of the oestrone-induced pituitary tumour.

The attractiveness of the "amphophilic" concept for the experimentally induced pituitary growth is that the tumours induced by totally different experimental procedures may be viewed as different aspects of the same phenomenon, all being "amphophilic tumours", and therefore not differing qualitatively but only quantitatively; i.e. the various subtypes of the "amphophilic" tumour produce different amounts of each of the pituitary hormones.

KONEFF, VAN DYKE and EVANS (1952) reported observations in parabiosis experiments indicating that an enhanced TSH and ACTH output resulted from the changes in the pituitary induced by thyroidectomy. CHAMORRO (1947) found changes in the mammary gland consisting of hypertrophy of the acini with secretion in the ducts in thyroidectomized rats and, to a lesser extent, also in rats treated with thyroid-blocking agents. Thus after the disruption of the thyroid-pituitary feed-back system as well as after oestrogen treatment the reported increase in hormonal functions does not appear to preclude the possibility that the functional changes induced in the pituitary differ only quantitatively; i.e. an increased output of most, if not all, hormones occurs in both cases, the difference being that after thyroid hormone deprivation the emphasis is on TSH-output, whereas after oestrogen treatment it is on prolactin-output.

B. 1. Discussion

BATES, CLIFTON and ANDERSON (1956) reported that prolactin could be found only in stilbestrol-induced and stilbestrol-dependent pituitary tumours of rats, and that it could not be detected in "dependent thyrotropic tumours" of mice, by the pigeon crop-gland method. The "thyrotropic tumours" were reported to contain very high amounts of TSH, whereas the stilbestrol-induced tumours contained little or no thyrotrophin, as assayed in baby chicks. Their findings are more in agreement with FURTH's concept of monohormonal pituitary tumours than with the view of potentially multihormonal "amphophilic" tumours, as developed above. It may be of interest to quote FURTH (1957) about this apparently equivocal output of prolactin output by the pituitary after thyroidectomy: "thyrotropes invariably have a trace of gonadotrophic activity, causing overproduction of oestrogens by the stimulated ovaries"; this hyperoestrogenization in its turn is thought to stimulate the "mammotropes" and thus the finding of stimulated mammary glands is accounted for.

The very model of FURTH's monomorphous, monohormonal pituitary tumour has therefore turned out, at least in the primary tumours induced in female mice to be one of a mixed cell population of "thyrotropes" and "mammotropes".

It should be noted that a slightly different interpretation of the facts might be that these "thyrotropic" tumours showed FSH- as well as prolactin-activity along with their high TSH-output.

It may be opportune to draw attention to a recent trend in the estimation of the physiological actions of the pituitary hormones, because the hypothesis that is suggested may form the theoretical basis of FURTH's attempt to reconcile his concept of a monomorphous and monohormonal pituitary tumour with experimental data suggestive of the action of more than one hormone.

ENGEL (1957) discussed some findings relating to common biological activities of several pituitary hormones and suggests as a possible explanation "common specific molecular configurations of peptide chains" in the very complex molecules of the different pituitary hormones. For the factual basis of this proposition he draws attention to "beta-MSH, which is a polypeptide with 18 amino acids and has in common with beta-corticotrophin a sequence of seven amino acids as well as two others close by. It seems altogether likely, as suggested by those who determined this structure (BELL and his collaborators) that "this sharing of amino acids accounts for the MSH activity of the corticotrophins, which has been such a puzzle in the past"; and ENGEL also draws attention to the even more striking example of alpha-MSH structure, elucidated by HARRIS and LEARNER (1957), which was found to have a sequence of 13 amino acids corresponding to those of beta-ACTH. It is apparently along similar lines that FURTH interpreted the gonadotrophic activities shown by the "thyrotropic" tumours since he states (FURTH, 1955, in the discussion following his paper): "On the basis of the constancy of some gonadotrophic stimulation by all (more than 10) thyrotropic tumour strains studied, I assume that this is not a "contamination" but a side effect of thyrotrophin manifest when this hormone is applied in large quantities, and is due to *some common or close chemical groups in the molecule* of thyrotrophin". Another example probably can be found in "the consistent occurrence of somatotropic changes with mammotrophic hormone activity in both female mice and rats with all mammotrophic tumour strains studied ...", which are ascribed not to an admixture of two types of cells or to two different hormones but to "*an inherent characteristic of one hormone* secreted by mammotropes ..." (FURTH, CLIFTON, GADSDEN and BUFFETT, 1956). It appears likely that this "inherent characteristic" is visualized also as "some common or close chemical group in the molecule" of prolactin and growth hormone.

The basis of the concept that the normal pituitary consists of six morphologically and functionally distinct cell types is the postulation of the existence of six separate and distinct hormones. From this concept the existence of monomorphous monohormonal pituitary tumours is inferred; when physiological evidence of hormonal activity of a supposedly monohormonal tumour, namely the changes induced in the host, is suggestive of more than one pituitary principle, the hypothesis is advanced that a pituitary hormone may have some structural characteristics in common with other pituitary hormones and that this may account for the observed changes in the host.

It appears that the last hypothesis undermines the very basis of the theory of monohormonal monomorphous tumours, i.e. the existence of separate and distinct pituitary hormones, which are characterized by the specific physiological actions that they induce. Even the purely hypothetical "common structural characteristics" of pituitary hormones may be interpreted to be more consistent with the earlier mentioned view of RIDDLE (page 11) that the "pituitary hormones" represent only "fragments" of the "true hormones", than with the view of six or more separate and distinct pituitary hormones and therefore may provide an interesting basis for the "multihormonal" pituitary cell concept. The final evaluation of these purely hypothetical interpretations of the experimental evidence must be postponed until the chemical structure of the hormones involved have been clarified. It serves to stress that a close link must be maintained between the study of the physiological action(s) as well as the other characteristics of pituitary hormones and the interpretation of the morphology of pituitary cells and of pituitary tumours. It should be appreciated that up to the present very little is known either about the exact chemical nature of the pituitary hormones as they exist in the gland or about their properties as they are secreted into the bloodstream and that it is not even certain that the biological activities reported for the purified hormones are necessarily those of the naturally secreted hormones because the chemist might inadvertently alter these hormones in his search for purity thereby eliminating some biological activities or even endowing the molecule with new properties, which nature did not intend it to have (ENGEL, 1957).

2. Summary and conclusions

The genetical constitution appears to influence the incidence of pituitary tumours in mice and rats; the other important factor in their formation seems to be the "hormonal balance" of the animal since a "hormonal imbalance" appears to be the distinctive feature common to most procedures that are followed by the development of pituitary tumors.

Depending on the view of the relationship between the morphologically different cells in the pituitary and their hormonal functions different concepts of the origin and nature of pituitary tumours are possible. The two extreme views are that pituitary tumours are derived from functionally and morphologically irreversibly differentiated, monohormonal cells; or pituitary tumours consist of "hormonally multipotent" cells. For the latter proposition two possibilities are considered; firstly the various cell types of the normal pituitary may be conceived as the various phases of one and the same cell so that all pituitary tumours are potentially capable of producing every hormone; or secondly "hormonally multipotent" cells may be conceived to exist along with the differentiated and functionally specialized cells in the normal pituitary, these "hormonally multipotent" cells proliferating and giving rise to pituitary tumours. This matter will be discussed in the light of the results of the present investigation.

The reciprocal regulatory action between the secretion of the hormones of the pituitary gland and the release of hormones by its target glands can be conceived to follow the pattern of "feed-back systems". FURTH and his collaborators suggest that the "hormonal imbalances" are the causative factor of pituitary tumours and that they can be divided into several types on the basis of the particular feed-back system disturbed. Consistent with his view of the monohormonal function of the various pituitary cell types, the induced pituitary tumours are divided into different types on the basis of the hormones secreted, which are presumed to indicate the feed-back system that was involved and the particular cell type induced to proliferate. This concept is very attractive because it seems to be concise and elegantly simple and to promise a new tool in the study of the nature of pituitary hormones by suggesting that "monohormonal monomorphous" masses of cells can be obtained. A survey of the data shows that a constant relationship between a well established type of "hormonal imbalance" and a definite functional type of pituitary tumour appears to be restricted to two types, namely that between hyperoestrogenization and prolactin-producing tumours and that between thyroid hormone deprivation and TSH-producing tumours. Some of the experimental data about both types of tumours require the additional hypothesis of "common chemical groups in the molecules" of some pituitary hormones to maintain the concept of monohormonal tumors and it is suggested that the relevant data may be considered to support equally well the multihormonal-cell concept.

A comparative study of the various characteristics of the two mentioned differently-induced types of pituitary tumours appears to be a useful approach to an assessment of the conflicting views about the nature and origin of pituitary tumours in general.

III. The incidence and the rate of growth of experimental pituitary tumours in various strains of mice

This chapter deals with the incidence and the rate of growth of pituitary tumours induced either by continuous oestrogen administration or by thyroid hormone deprivation in rats and mice.

One of the disputed questions is whether the differently induced pituitary tumours have something more in common than the mere fact that they occur in the pituitary gland. It has been suggested that the induction mechanisms may have a "common pathway"; i.e. the various hormonal derangements either have a common factor, which is responsible for the induction of tumourous growth in the pituitary, or they act on the same cell type, (see page 17, II. 4. a. and page 18, II. 4. b. respectively). If such a common pathway exists it will probably manifest itself in some of the biological characteristics of the tumours. GORBMAN (1956) has drawn attention to the possible significance of the fact that the $C_{57}Bl$ strain of mice appears to be the one, which most readily yields pituitary tumours after oestrogen treatment as well as after destruction of the thyroid gland by radioactive iodine. An assessment of the influence of the genetic constitution on the one hand and of the type of hormonal imbalance on the other on the incidence and on the growth rate of experimental pituitary tumours appeared to offer a useful approach to an opinion on the disputed existence of a common pathway. Special attention was given to the question whether an identical sequence could be found for the two totally different hormonal derangements, oestrogen excess and thyroid hormone deficiency, when the various strains of mice included into the investigation were arranged according to their liability to develop pituitary tumours or to the rate of growth of their tumours.

The data from the literature are not suggestive of a "parallelism" between the incidences of oestrone-induced and of "radiothyroidectomy"-induced pituitary tumours in mice and rats. The well established difference in the incidence of oestrogen-induced pituitary tumours in various strains of mice appear to be in contrast to the reported high incidence in all strains investigated after destruction of the thyroid gland by radioactive iodine (see II. 2. a.). In rats oestrogen administration has been proved effective beyond doubt in producing pituitary tumours, whereas thyroid hormone deprivation in this respect must be considered by far inferior to oestrogen treatment, if it is effective at all (see II. 2. b.). The difficulty of comparing the reported pituitary tumour incidences obtained with different experimental procedures in different laboratories is obvious and a comparative study of pituitary tumours induced in one and the same laboratory by the two hormonal derangements appeared to be desirable.

Prof. Mühlbock has been so kind as to permit access to data and materials concerning the pituitaries of experiments in the Netherland's Cancer Institute covering a period of more than six years. Data on the incidence of pituitary adenomata in mice as a result of long term treatment with oestrone have mostly been derived from experiments performed to ascertain the effect of oestrone on the mammary tumour incidence in various strains. Data on pituitary adenoma induction by the thyroid-blocking agent methylthiouracil have come from experiments set up primarily to study thyroid tumours. All experiments with rats and the experiments using radioactive iodine to destroy the thyroid glands in mice were planned to study pituitary tumours.

A. Experimental

1. Materials and methods

a) Animals: Four highly-inbred strains of mice: $C_{57}Bl$; O_{20}; CBA and C_3H_f and two F_1-hybrids: $C_{57}Bl \times DBA_f$ and $O_{20} \times DBA_f$ and the highly-inbred strain of rats, R-Amsterdam, have been studied.

The mice were kept in glass cages of $17 \times 11 \times 12$ cm, four to a cage unless otherwise stated; the rats were kept in metal cages of $29 \times 22 \times 16$ cm, three to a cage.

The diet for mice consisted, unless otherwise stated, of commercial food pellets (Laboratoriumratten korrels verrijkt met soja en vitamine D; ROEST's Pluimvee- en Veevoederfabriek, Heemstede, Holland) and tap water continuously available ad libitum. In addition, twice weekly a handful of whole wheat was provided per cage. The diet for rats consisted of commercial food pellets (Konijnen korrels, ROEST's Pluimvee- en Veevoederfabriek, Heemstede, Holland) and tap water continuously available ad libitum and in addition fresh lettuce and meat offal, i.e. rumen etc. were provided twice weekly.

b) Method of administration of the drugs used. For these experiments the natural oestrogen *oestrone* has been used. This was dissolved in drinking water for the experiments with mice (BOOT and MÜHLBOCK, 1956). A dose of 125 μg of oestrone per litre of drinking water is just sufficient to cause constant vaginal oestrus in ovariectomized mice and the oestrone dose reaching the general circulation presumably corresponds with the average oestrogen production in intact females, or is somewhat below it. The dose used for pituitary tumour induction, corresponding with the maximal solubility of oestrone in water, was 2,000 μg per litre. A fresh solution of oestrone in drinking water was prepared once weekly by adding 1 mil. of a stock solution (400 mg of oestrone dissolved in 100 mil. C_2H_5OH) to a litre of tap water.

The efficacy of oestrone given to mice in their drinking water may be due to a sufficient amount of oestrogen by-passing the liver owing to absorption through portions of the alimentary canal or in some other way or it might be due to an overwhelming of the liver's capacity to degrade oestrogen so that unchanged oestrogen reaches the general circulation. Both these mechanisms may operate. In rats apparently these mechanisms do not allow sufficient amounts of oestrone to reach the general circulation as even the 2,000 μg per litre dose of oestrone in drinking water proved not always sufficient to induce constant vaginal oestrus in ovariectomized rats (BOOT, personal communication). Therefore the method of choice of oestrone administration in rats has been the sub-cutaneous implantation of pellets. Appropriate amounts of oestrone and cholesterol (weight ratio 1 to 3) were mixed by dissolving in benzene, whereupon the solvens was evaporated under a hood; the resulting homogenous dry mixture was compressed into pellets of approximately 2 mg (diameter 1.1 mm, length approximately 3 mm). One pellet was implanted weekly into each rat.

Methylthiouracil was given in foodpellets containing 0.4% of the drug. Commercial foodpellets were ground into fine powder, to each kilogram 4 gram of methylthiouracil was added, thoroughly mixed and the resulting mixture was reconstituted into pellets. The diet of the experimental animals consisted exclusively of these pellets, and tap water was available ad libitum.

Thyroxin was administered in drinking water, the dose being 6 mg per litre of tap water. A stock solution was made by dissolving 60 mg of thyroxin in 10 mil. 0.1 N NaOH. The stock solution was kept in the dark at 4° C and every other week a fresh stock solution was prepared.

Thyroxinized drinking water was made by adding 1 mil. of the stock solution to 1 l of tap water, the NaOH was neutralized by finally adding 1 mil. of 0.1 N HCl. The thyroxinized drinking water was renewed twice weekly. With this regimen it was possible to prevent goitrous changes in mice receiving methylthiouracil. The method of administration has the slight draw-back that some strains develop an enhanced diuresis after a certain period and it may be necessary to readjust the thyroxin concentration to assure a constant intake of hormone.

Radioactive iodine was administered as a single intra-peritoneal dose of a sterile, isotonic aqueous solution of $Na^{131}I$, the ph being adjusted to 8—9. The dose for mice was standardized at 0.2 mil. and for rats at 1.0 mil. The animals were put on a low iodine diet, consisting exclusively of whole wheat and distilled water for a period of ten days, beginning 7 days prior to the administration of radioactive iodine.

The standardization of the amount of radioactive iodine has been based on the assumption that a concentration of approximately 4 μC per mg of gland be considered the minimum thyroid-destructive dose (GORBMAN, 1950). The percentage of the administered dose of radioactive iodine recovered from the thyroid gland 24 hrs after the administration gives a fair approximation to the maximum concentration that is reached in the gland. Experiments with tracer doses of ^{131}I showed that the 24 hrs "uptake" of radioactive iodine by the thyroids had a range of 16% to 48%. The differences were suggestive of strain differences in thyroid activity but the number of mice of the different strains was not sufficient for statistical evaluation. The weights of the thyroid in mice of the various strains, killed at the age of 10 to 14 weeks, did not show large differences and were approximately 4 mg. The results indicate that a dose of 200 μC intraperitoneally may be expected to be a reliable thyroid-destructive dose even in mice with a low ^{131}I uptake by the thyroid. Since it has been suggested that radiation is an important contributory factor in pituitary tumourigenesis after destruction of the thyroid gland by radioactive iodine (GORBMAN, 1956; see II. 4. b., page 17) the advantage of using the same dose of ^{131}I in all strains of mice thus exposing them to approximately the same dose of whole body irradiation is obvious when one objective of the experiments is to evaluate strain differences in the liability to develop pituitary tumours after hormonal derangements.

The minimum thyroid-destructive dose of radioactive iodine for rats was calculated from the mean 24 hrs "uptake" of a tracer dose of ^{131}I and the mean thyroid weights at the age of 60 to 90 days to be approximately 600 μC it being assumed that the radiation sensitivity of thyroid tissue is of the same order in rats as in mice. In a pilot experiment increasing doses of ^{131}I were injected into 5 groups of rats, each group comprising 2 males and 2 females. The rats of the first, the second, the third, the fourth and the fifth group received 450 μC, 550 μC, 675 μC, 800 μC and 1000 μC respectively. All rats were sacrificed after 10 weeks. Microscopical examination of the thyroid region showed that total destruction had been achieved in the groups that received 800 μC or more.

Check on thyroid destruction: The trachea and its overlying musculature including the whole thyroid gland region were removed from the first twenty mice given ^{131}I and serially sectioned at 4 μ. One out of every ten sections was examined microscopically for residual thyroid tissue. Only hyalinized or calcified scar-tissue was found, the bloodvessels in the neighbourhood showing the characteristic thickening. Only occasionally a few cells, which may have been epithelial remnants of the thyroid gland were seen within this scar-tissue. They did not show any tendency to follicle formation and it is doubtful whether they have any functional significance. This laborious check was subsequently performed on only four or five animals chosen at random from each new injection series. In addition, the thyroid glands from all mice without the expected pituitary tumour at the time of autopsy were examined microscopically. Independently of this microscopical verification a tracer dose of 10 μC was injected into a few series of mice 6 to 8 months after the injection of the 200 μC dose and the radioactivity over the neck region was compared with the radioactivity over the thigh region on the day following the administration of the tracer dose. No signs of residual thyroid activity were ever found, whereas regeneration of a few follicles were sometimes found microscopically months later at the time of autopsy in a few of the mice without pituitary tumours.

In rats thyroid destruction was checked microscopically as in mice, except that only one out of every fifty 4 μ sections were examined from the whole region; one out of every 5 sections were examined of the region of the isthmus, the most caudal and the most rostral parts of the gland, these being the regions in which regeneration most likely occurs. All the rats from the pilot experiment were examined in this way. In the following eight "routineseries" only five animals randomly chosen from each series were so examined. Analysis of the data at the end of the experiment showed that the precautions taken to assure thyroid destruction in the rats had not been sufficient. Although all the rats injected in the first as well as in the last two series may be considered to have received an adequate dose of radioactive iodine, the thyroid glands of all the randomly selected animals from these groups showing only scar-tissue, in the 5 series comprising the rats injected in the period from June 1955 until August 1956 and consisting of 110 rats (males and females) the injections had failed to eliminate the thyroid gland. The sections from these series showed thyroid remnants, ranging from practically normal-appearing gland to fibrous scar-tissue in which a few colloid-containing follicles enmeshed in connective tissue fibres could be found located especially in the periphery of the scar. Another group of 20 male rats was injected with 2,000 μC per rat and the result of this dose of radioactive iodine was checked microscopically in each rat at the time of autopsy.

c) **Method of classification of pituitary glands.** Evaluation of the results of the various hormonal derangements on the pituitary in rats as well as in mice was based on the weight of the pituitary at the time of autopsy. The pituitaries were classified as "normal", "adenomateously enlarged" or as "tumours" according to the observed weight.

A maximum weight limit was defined for "normal" and a minimum weight limit for "tumours", the pituitaries having a weight above the limit for "normal", but still below that for "tumours" being considered "adenomateously enlarged". For mice the minimum weight limit for pituitary tumours of 12 mg has been used by GARDNER (1941) and has been adopted here. For rats a weight of 30 mg as used by CLIFTON and MEYER (1956 b) has been adopted as the minimum limit for pituitary tumours. The maximum weight limit for "normal" pituitaries was arbitrarily set for mice at 3 mg and for rats at 12 mg. Since the "time factor" influences the weight that the pituitaries attain, the available data have been divided into several periods according to the duration of the hormonal imbalance at the time of autopsy.

2. Results:

a) In mice. The results of classifying the pituitaries of the various strains of mice that have been subjected to a thyroid-destructive dose of radioactive iodine and to continuous oestrone administration are given in Table 3. The pituitary weights after methylthiouracil treatment and those after the combined oestrone and methylthiouracil treatment were available for three of the strains and are included in Table 3.

In most of the strains investigated, oestrone treatment and "radiothyroidectomy" appear to be equally effective in inducing pituitary tumours. The C_{57}Bl strain and the F_1-hybrids appear to yield pituitary tumours in a very high incidence. When the "time factor" is taken into consideration, it becomes evident that mice of the C_{57}Bl strain yield pituitary tumours most readily irrespective of the type of hormonal derangement; pituitary tumours are already found at an early period (200—300 days) and the peak of the recorded pituitary tumours, which reflects to some extent the time needed for the tumours to attain a size that is incompatible with life owing to "cerebral compression", is around 400 days of treatment. By these criteria the (C_{57}Bl $\times$ DBA$_f$) F_1-hybrid and the (O_{20} $\times$ DBA$_f$) F_1-hybrid mice come second and third respectively, for both the oestrone-induced and the „radiothyroidectomy"-induced tumours. In the O_{20}-, the CBA- and the C_3H_f-strains, the earliest pituitary tumours occur definitely later (400—500 days of treatment). The data on "radiothyroidectomy"-induced pituitary tumours in the two first mentioned strains are not beyond reproach. In the O_{20} strain it is doubtful whether total destruction of the thyroid gland was achieved in all mice, since in 7 out of 20 C_{57}Bl mice from the same injection series (18. 9. 1953) thyroid remnants with signs of hyperactivity were found on microscopic examination of the trachea. Accidentally the thyroid regions of the O_{20} mice were not kept for microscopic examination. The lower incidences in the "radiothyroidectomy" group (6 out of 10 mice surviving the treatment for more than 400 but less than 500 days and 9 out of 16 mice surviving more than 500 days) as compared with the corresponding oestrone groups (4 out of 5 mice and 19 out of 20 mice respectively) reflect a greater dispersion in the pituitary weights in the „thyroidectomy" group, due, possibly, to thyroid regeneration in some of the mice. The

Table 3. *Classification of pituitaries according to weight for six strains of mice subjected to treatment leading to tumourous enlargement of the pituitaries*[1]

Strain	Days after initiation of treatment	Treatment groups: Oestrone n./e./t.[2]	Na^{131}I n./e./t.	MTU n./e./t.	MTU + oestrone n./e./t.
C_{57}Bl	200—300	0. 2. 8.	0. 0. 3.	0. 3. 0.	1. 12. 3.
	300—400	0. 2. 10.	0. 0. 5.	3. 5. 4.	0. 9. 9.
	400—500	0. 1. 19.	0. 0. 7.	5. 7. 3.	0. 0. 1.
	500 and more	0. 0. 0.	0. 0. 5.	7. 5. 6.	0. 2. 0.
C_3Hf	200—300	117. 0. 0.	11. 6. 0.		
	300—400	83. 2. 0.	2. 4. 1.		
	400—500	40. 0. 0.	0. 0. 3.		
	500 and more	19. 0. 0.	0. 0. 0.		
CBA	200—300	1. 0. 0.	6. 0. 0.		
	300—400	22. 0. 0.	2. 0. 0.		
	400—500	16. 2. 2.	0. 0. 0.		
	500 and more	11. 6. 11.	1. 0. 1.		
O_{20}	200—300	0. 0. 0.	1. 0. 0.		
	300—400	0. 1. 0.	0. 0. 0.		
	400—500	0. 1. 4.	0. 4. 6.		
	500 and more	0. 1. 19.	0. 7. 9.		
(C_{57}Bl × DBAf)F_1	200—300	0. 0. 0.	0. 1. 0.	1. 0. 0.	0. 0. 0.
	300—400	0. 0. 9.	0. 3. 7.	1. 0. 1.	2. 6. 11.
	400—500	2. 3. 27.	0. 1. 52.	7. 3. 1.	1. 10. 11.
	500 and more	0. 3. 29.	0. 0. 18.	25. 27. 4.	0. 11. 24.
(O_{20} × DBAf)F_1	200—300	0. 2. 0.	1. 1. 0.	2. 0. 0.	4. 6. 0.
	300—400	1. 0. 5.	0. 0. 2.	7. 8. 0.	6. 8. 1.
	400—500	0. 7. 51.	0. 8. 4.	1. 10. 3.	1. 2. 1.
	500 and more	0. 8. 84.	0. 10. 32.	5. 18. 15.	4. 13. 1.

[1] Pituitary weight data of males, orchidectomized males, females and spayed females in the different strains of mice have been pooled.

[2] n. = number of pituitaries weighing 3 mg or less, considered "normal".
e. = number of pituitaries weighing between 3 mg and 12 mg, considered "enlarged".
t. = number of pituitaries weighing 12 mg or more, considered "tumourously enlarged".

times of occurrence of pituitary tumours as well as the times needed by the tumours to attain comparable sizes are of approximately the same magnitude in the two treatment groups. In the CBA strain the intercurrent mortality in the "radiothyroidectomy" group was extremely high and only two animals survived longer than 400 days after starting treatment; one pituitary tumour was observed and this suggests that destruction of the thyroid gland by radioactive iodine ultimately may result in the development of pituitary tumours in this strain too, since spontaneous pituitary tumours are extremely rare in mice except when genetic factors favour their occurrence. Although the number of observations does not justify the conclusion that the incidence and the time of occurrence in the two treatment groups of this strain run parallel, it can be stated that the experimental data are not in disagreement with this proposition. The more striking therefore is the behaviour of the C_3H strain. It is impossible to test the efficacy of oestrone in this strain when the milk factor is present since the mice succumb to mammary tumours before any pituitary tumour can be expected to develop. Mice of the C_3H_f and C_3H_e having the same genetic constitution but without the milk agent survive long enough for pituitary tumours to develop after adequate hormonal derangement as the "radiothyroidectomy" series demonstrates. One of the seven mice examined 300—400 days after the administration of ^{131}I and all three that survived more than 400 days had tumours. By contrast after comparable periods of oestrone administration no tumours developed in 85 and 59 mice respectively. It can therefore be stated that mice of the C_3H genetic constitution are completely resistant to continuous oestrone administration, although "radiothyroidectomy" induces pituitary tumours in them. The inability of oestrone to induce pituitary enlargement is the more striking as demonstrated by the fact that only two pituitaries weighed more than 3 mg out of the 144 mice autopsied 300 or more days after the initiation of the oestrone regimen, these two pituitaries weighing only 3.4 and 4.0 mg respectively.

In comparison with thyroid destruction by radioactive iodine methylthiouracil treatment is far inferior in inducing pituitary tumours in the three strains of mice; the pituitary weights obtained after methylthiouracil were less than after "radiothyroidectomy" and/or the tumours tended to become manifest after a longer time interval. This is in agreement with the results described by others (Gorbman, 1956; Dent, Gadsden and Furth, 1956, etc.).

The pituitary enlargement resulting from combined treatment of mice with oestrone and methylthiouracil was not as pronounced as after oestrone alone. This appears to be in agreement with observations on rats (Gillman and Gilbert, 1955). Thus it appears that methylthiouracil inhibits the induction of pituitary tumours by oestrone. It may be presumed that this effect of methylthiouracil is due to the depression of metabolism caused by thyroid hormone deprivation. According to Dent, Gadsden and Furth (1956) the difference between the effects of methylthiouracil treatment and „radiothyroidectomy" on pituitary tumourigenesis is accounted for by the different degrees of thyroid hormone deficiency produced by the two methods; after thyroid gland destruction it is complete, whereas after chemical "blocking" of the hormone synthesis a "leak" is presumed to occur. The relatively greater effectiveness of methylthiouracil, approaching that of "radiothyroidectomy" in inducing pituitary tumours in the ($O_{20} \times DBA_f$) F_1-hybrids may be attributable to a more effective blocking of hormone synthesis in these hybrids than in the two other strains. This view apparently is supported by the finding that methylthiouracil lowers the pituitary tumour inducing effect of oestrone most pronouncedly in these particular hybrids.

In Table 4 the effect of various treatments and some combinations of treatments on pituitary weights in castrated male ($C_{57}Bl \times DBA_f$) F_1 hybrids mice are given. The results demonstrate again that both oestrone treatment and "radiothyroidectomy" are very effective in inducing pitui-

Table 4. *Classification of pituitaries according to weight for* $(C_{57}Bl \times DBA_f)F_1$, *orchidectomized male mice subjected to different treatments*

Days after initiation of treatment	Treatment groups					
	Oestrone	$Na^{131}I$	MTU	Oestrone + $Na^{131}I$	Oestrone + MTU	$Na^{131}I$ + thyroxin
	n./e./t.[1]	n./e./t.	n./e./t.	n./e./t.	n./e./t.	n./e./t.
200—300	0. 0. 0.	0. 0. 0.	0. 0. 0.	0. 0. 0.	0. 0. 0.	1. 0. 0.
300—400	0. 0. 7.	0. 2. 0.	2. 0. 0.	0. 1. 7.	2. 2. 0.	1. 0. 0.
400—500	0. 0. 7.	0. 0. 11.	0. 2. 0.	0. 0. 6.	1. 2. 3.	14. 0. 0.
500 and more	0. 0. 1.	0. 0. 3.	1. 11. 3.	0. 0. 0.	0. 1. 3.	0. 0. 0.

[1] n. = number of pituitaries weighing 3 mg or less, considered "normal".
e. = number of pituitaries weighing between 3 mg and 12 mg, considered "enlarged".
t. = number of pituitaries weighing 12 mg or more, considered "tumourously enlarged".

tary tumours. The apparent difference between them is due to the method of classification of the pituitaries. The complete preventive action of continuous thyroxin administration is clearly demonstrated and is in agreement with the results of GOLDBERG and CHAIKOFF (1951). Again the superiority of "radiothyroidectomy" over methylthiouracil administration in inducing pituitary tumours is clearly demonstrated, but, whereas methylthiouracil in combination with oestrone prolongs the induction time and lowers the incidence of pituitary tumours as compared with oestrone alone, the results of "radiothyroidectomy" in combination with continuous oestrone administration shows no appreciable difference as compared with oestrone administration alone. This invalidates the proposed hypothesis that the pituitary tumour retarding effect of methylthiouracil in mice is connected with its thyroid hormone depriving action. Since the mice on a methylthiouracil regimen have significantly lower body weights than either the oestrone-treated or the "radiothyroidectomized" mice, the retarding effect was thought to be due to restricted caloric intake.

To rule out any contributory effect of its thyroid hormone depriving action on the retardation of the development of pituitary tumours, the effect of methylthiouracil on pituitary tumour induction by a thyroid-destructive dose of radioactive iodine was investigated. Castrated male $C_{57}Bl$ mice were divided into four groups; the mice in group A were put on the methylthiouracil regimen, and those in group B, C and D were injected with a thyroid-destructive dose of ^{131}I, but the mice in group B were fed the normal diet ad libitum, those in group C were fed methylthiouracil pellets ad libitum and those of group D were put one to a cage and received a restricted amount of normal food (pellets and whole grain) daily. The amount of food received daily by group D was adjusted in an effort to keep the body weights of the mice matched to the body weights of the mice in group C. The body weights were controlled weekly. During the first four weeks, however, it was impossible to restrict the food sufficiently to keep the body weights matched closely, without killing the animals in group D. During this period the mean body weight of the animals in group D was allowed to exceed that of group C by approximately two grams.

The results of the experiment are given in Table 5. The pituitary weights demonstrate a significant retardation of the growth of pituitary tumours induced by a thyroid-destructive dose of radioactive iodine if it is combined with methylthiouracil. This retardation appears to be equalled by that caused by a restriction of the food intake. It is proposed that reduced caloric intake (and/or utilisation) can account for the retarding effect of methylthiouracil on pituitary enlargement. Since the reduced caloric intake may be presumed also to retard pituitary tumour development induced by methylthiouracil, the superiority of "radiothyroidectomy" over methylthiouracil treatment may be partly attributed to this cause. The fact that combined "radiothyroidectomy" and methylthiouracil

Table 5. *The effect on pituitary-, adrenal- and thymic weight of methylthiouracil treatment, destruction of the thyroid gland by* ^{131}I, *the combination of both treatments and the combination of „radiothyroidectomy" and restriction of food intake in castrated male* $C_{57}Bl$ *mice. (10 months after initiation of treatment)*

Group	Number of animals	Treatment	Weight in mg ± standard error, the range is given in parentheses		
			pituitary	adrenals	thymus
A	11	methylthiouracil-food pellets and tapwater ad lib.	4.0± 0.87 (1.8—11.1)	3.4±0.22 (1.8—4.3)	32.5±2.29 (26.5—48.0)
B	4	"radiothyroidectomy" normal foodpellets and tapwater ad lib.	54.1±12.15 (34.2—76.1)	4.3±0.33 (3.4—4.7)	26.1± 6.92 (8.0—37.1)
C	11	"radiothyroidectomy" methylthiouracil-food-pellets and tapwater ad lib.	14.2± 3.74 (4.7—50.1)	3.0±0.19 (2.2—3.8)	28.0± 2.29 (11.1—35.9)
D	11	"radiothyroidectomy" restricted intake of normal foodpellets, tapwater ad lib.	16.8± 2.72 (7.0—37.0)	4.2±0.24 (3.5—6.3)	10.5± 1.93 (3.6—23.8)

For intergroup comparison the statistical significance (p) for each comparable pair was calculated[1] to be:

Pituitary weight: $A < B$: $p < 0.01$; $A < C$: $0.01 < p < 0.02$; $A < D$: $p < 0.01$; $B > C$: $p < 0.01$; $B > D$: $p < 0.01$; $C < D$: $0.60 < p < 0.70$.

Adrenal weight: $A < B$: $0.02 < p < 0.05$; $A > C$: $0.10 < p < 0.20$; $A < D$: $0.02 < p < 0.05$; $B > C$: $p < 0.01$; $B > D$: $0.80 < p < 0.90$; $C < D$: $p < 0.01$.

thymic weight: $A > B$: $0.20 < p < 0.30$; $A > C$: $0.10 < p < 0.20$; $A > D$: $p < 0.01$; $B < C$: $0.70 < p < 0.80$; $B > D$: $p < 0.01$; $C > D$: $p < 0.01$.

[1] Student's t-test.

treatment is more effective than the latter alone, however, clearly demonstrates that there must be an additional factor responsible for the difference. It seems improbable that the additional factor depends on a difference in the degree of stimulation of the pituitary to produce TSH, since the TSH-assays (see chapter V.B. 3.b) indicated that after methylthiouracil treatment the increase of the TSH content of the pituitary is of the same order as after "radiothyroidectomy". At least in the period when the pituitary mass has not yet increased appreciably, both procedures lead to an increase of TSH that is probably maximal. It is therefore suggested that this "additional factor" should be ascribed to the irradiation by ^{131}I to which the "radiothyroidectomy" mice are subjected (GORBMAN, 1956).

The extremely low thymic weights in the "radiothyroidectomized" mice with restricted food intake suggest an enhanced corticoid output by the adrenals. It seems that the pituitary of a "radiothyroidectomized" mouse can respond to the "stress" of food restriction by a continuously increasing ACTH-output and that the pituitaries of such mice on a normal diet are not subjected to an increased demand for ACTH as has been suggested (EDELMANN, 1955). Since the proposition has been made that after oestrone treatment and "radiothyroidectomy" respectively an increased demand for one pituitary hormone alone, namely prolactin or TSH may not be sufficient to induce pituitary tumour development although an increased demand for two pituitary hormones may do so (EDELMANN, 1955; GORBMAN, 1956), it may be of interest to pose the question whether the "reduced caloric intake" in the present experiments retards pituitary tumour development through a general depression of metabolism or by imposing an increased demand for ACTH as well as an increased demand for TSH in "the radiothyroidectomized" mice.

The normal thymic weights in both groups of mice on the methylthiouracil regimen indicate that the output of adrenal corticoids could not have been enhanced significantly by the presumed "reduced caloric intake". Although the thymic weights do not suggest an enhanced output of pituitary ACTH, such an enhanced output induced by the "stress" of "reduced caloric intake" cannot be excluded, since the low adrenal weights in these groups may reflect the reported inability of the adrenals in most strains of mice treated with methylthiouracil to respond to ACTH (CASAS and KOPPISCH, 1952) and thus the unimpaired thymic weights may be accounted for.

b) In rats. The results of classifying the pituitaries of rats of various treatment groups and of untreated rats are given in Table 6.

Compared with most other strains reported (see II. I. b.), rats of the R-Amsterdam strain have a relatively low incidence of spontaneous pituitary tumours. The incidence obviously increases with age and amongst animals from the breeder colony that are kept to a very old age of more than 1000 days, the incidence has risen to over 60%. Since the duration of treatment is considered more relevant to the pituitary tumour incidence than the actual age of the rats and most experimental animals were at the age of 2 to 3 months at the start of the experiments, 75 days have been deducted from the actual age of the control rats so as to allocate them to the various periods of "duration of treatment". In 91 untreated rats only 3 pituitary tumours were found, all occurring in the last two age groups. When compared with this control group it is clearly demonstrated that only the rats treated with oestrone showed a definite effect on pituitary tumour development. Thyroxin treatment possibly has a slight enhancing effect on pituitary tumour development in rats, since in the thyroxin treated animals pituitary tumours were seen earlier than in the untreated rats. Moreover thyroxin treatment combined with oestrone treatment yielded slightly larger pituitary tumours at corresponding ages than oestrone treatment alone. Contrary to this, thyroid hormone deprivation by successful destruction of the thyroid gland by radioactive iodine had a distinct retarding effect on the tumour development induced by oestrone.

Microscopic examination of the trachea and its muscles, including the whole thyroid region, showed that in five series of radioactive iodine administrations the radiation delivered to the thyroid gland had not been sufficient to destroy it totally. The majority of the rats that were "radiothyroidectomized" only and all the rats that received thyroxin in their drinking water in addition, belonged to these five series; all the rats, which received oestrone treatment in addition were of the two last series and showed only scar tissue in the thyroid region.

The microscopic appearance of the pituitaries as well as of the thyroid remnants of the rats of the series that did not receive an adequate thyroid-destructive dose of radioactive iodine indicated that the thyroid-pituitary feed-back mechanism had been disturbed. Typical "thyroidectomy" cells were present in almost all pituitaries of rats in the groups injected with radioactive iodine alone; the thyroid remnants also showed evidence of a disturbed thyroid-pituitary feed-back since they often contained large cells with a "foamy" cytoplasm, forming small follicles that contained little or no colloid and sometimes the cells were not even arranged in follicular structure but in compact cell rows. For the pituitary weight data of the "radiothyroidectomized" series in Table 6 only those rats have been taken into consideration that showed one or both of the following indications of severe thyroid hormone deprivation namely the finding of extensive scar tissue with only a few regenerated follicles and the absence of granulated acidophile cells in the pituitary. The findings suggest that thyroid hormone deprivation retards the development of pituitary tumours, since the only two pituitaries that attained a size classified as "tumourous" weighed only 30.6 mg and 31.8 mg, whereas the smallest spontaneous pituitary tumour weighed over 110 mg and the two others more than 200 mg. It should be mentioned, that in the group of rats that received a 1000 μC dose of radioactive iodine but in which the thyroid gland showed only slight damage at the time of autopsy, there was one pituitary tumour weighing 220 mg. This tumour was found in a castrated male rat 663 days after the administration of radioactive iodine; the pituitary tumour consisted of large cells with vesicular nuclei and prominent nucleoli. The cytoplasm stained pale blue in the Mallory trichrome modification and appeared devoid of granules. The thyroid gland showed no appreciable residual signs of radiation damage except for a slight increase of interfollicular connective tissue. The thyroid gland did not show any sign of excessive pituitary stimulation; the follicles were large, contained normal-appearing colloid and were lined with "flattened-cuboidal" epithelium; neither the cytoplasm nor the nuclei of the cells gave the impression of enhanced physiological activity. It appears therefore justifiable to consider this pituitary tumour to be a chromophobe adenoma, which developed spontaneously, there being no causal relationship between it and the administration of a dose of radioactive iodine that proved grossly inadequate to destroy the thyroid gland.

The results of the combined treatment with radioactive iodine and continuous thyroxin administration permit the conclusion that the amount of "whole body irradiation" resulting from the administration of 1000 μC of radioactive iodine, does not materially affect the pituitary tumour incidence.

The results of oestrone treatment alone, when compared to the combined oestrone and thyroid treatment on the one hand and oestrone administration after successful "radiothyroidectomy" on the other, suggest that thyroid hormone deficiency retards pituitary tumour development, whereas excess of thyroid hormone possibly enhances it. In the untreated, the "radiothyroidectomized" and the thyroxin-treated groups the results are suggestive of a parallel situation: thyroid hormone deficiency possibly retards pituitary tumour development and the tumours are smaller,

Table 6. *Classification of pituitaries according to weight for rats, strain R-Amsterdam, subjected to different treatments*[1]

Days after initiation of treatment[2]	Treatment groups						
	oestrone	$Na^{131}I$[3]	thyroxin	control	oestrone + $Na^{131}I$	oestrone + thyroxin	$Na^{131}I$ + thyroxin
	n./e./t.[4]	n./e./t.	n./e./t.	n./e./t.	n./e./t.	n./e./t.	n./e./t.
75—150	0. 3. 6.	0. 0. 0.	7. 0. 0.	0. 0. 0.	2. 13. 0.	0. 3. 7.	0. 0. 0.
150—300	0. 0. 16[5]	0. 1. 0.	7. 2. 0.	5. 0. 0.	0. 1. 0.	0. 0. 15.[6]	1. 1. 0.
300—450	0. 0. 0.	4. 1. 0.	1. 0. 0.	27. 7. 0.	1. 1. 14.	0. 0. 0.	2. 0. 0.
450—600	0. 0. 0.	0. 2. 0.	2. 3. 2.	24. 0. 0.	0. 0. 1.	0. 0. 0.	5. 4. 0.
600—750	0. 0. 0.	8. 9. 0.	0. 3. 1.	12. 2. 1.	0. 0. 0.	0. 0. 0.	4. 9. 1.
750—900	0. 0. 0.	3. 9. 2.[7]	0. 0. 0.	4. 7. 2.	0. 0. 0.	0. 0. 0.	0. 2. 0.

[1] Pituitary weight data of males, orchidectomized males, females and spayed females in the different treatment groups have been pooled.

[2] "Duration of treatment" for the untreated rats = actual age — 75 days.

[3] Administration of radioactive iodine in this group of rats resulted in an incomplete destruction of the thyroid gland in the majority of animals (see text).

[4] n. = number of pituitaries weighing 12 mg or less, considered "normal".
e. = number of pituitaries weighing between 12 mg and 30 mg, considered "enlarged".
t. = number of pituitaries weighing 30 mg or more, considered "tumourously enlarged".

[5] Mean tumour weight: 117 mg; range: 77 mg — 195 mg. (150 days to 170 days).

[6] Mean tumour weight: 205 mg; range: 179 mg — 309 mg. (150 days to 170 days).

[7] The actual weight of these two pituitaries were respectively 30.6 and 31.8 mg.

whereas thyroid hormone excess possibly has an enhancing action since the tumours are observed earlier than in the untreated rats. Although "radiothyroidectomy" has been proved incomplete in 30 out of the 39 rats included in the "radiothyroidectomy" group inTable 6, the results suggest that contrary to the situation in mice, rats of the R-Amsterdam strain are resistant to pituitary tumour induction by "radiothyroidectomy". This is in agreement with the negative results mentioned by FURTH, DENT, BURNETT and GADSDEN (1955) in rats, which were claimed to have been "adequately radiothyroidectomized".

Table 7. *Classification of pituitaries according to weight for 17 completely radiothyroidectomized (histologically verified) male strain R-Amsterdam rats (injected dose 2 mC ^{131}I)*

Days after initiation of treatment	n./e./t.[1]	Pituitary weights in mg	
		mean	range
300—450	3. 0. 0.	10.2	10.0—10.4
450—600	0. 3. 0.	14.2	13.0—15.7
600—750	1. 10. 0.	14.3	11.7—16.8

[1] Same as in Table 6.

Since it appeared important to give this negative conclusion a sound basis a new series of rats, exclusively males, were injected with 2000 μC of radioactive iodine. The whole thyroid region of each rat was serially sectioned and examined microscopically at the end of the experiment and only data from the rats that were shown to have a totally destroyed thyroid gland without any sign of regeneration of thyroid tissue are included in Table 7.

B. Discussion and conclusions

The experiments reveal a remarkable contrast between the reactions of C_3H_f mice and R-Amsterdam rats. In C_3H_f mice oestrone fails to induce pituitary tumours although "radiothyroidectomy" is effective; in R-Amsterdam rats oestrone effectively induces pituitary tumours whereas "radiothyroidectomy" does not. The opposite results can be explained most readily by assuming that the "mammotropes" of the C_3H_f mice and the "thyrotropes" of the rats are resistant to continuous and specific stimulation and do not react thereto by unrestricted proliferation. These results thus appear to be more consistent with FURTH's concept of the origin and nature of pituitary tumours (see II. 4. a.) than with a "common pathway", but the results in the five other strains of mice lead to a different conclusion. In these strains both types of hormonal derangement induce tumourous enlargement and with equal efficiency. In particular the close parallelism between the results of oestrone treatment and "radiothyroidectomy" in the C_{57}Bl strain and in the two F_1-hybrids (C_{57}Bl $\times$ DBA_f) and (O_{20} $\times$ DBA_f) is very striking: not only is the sequence the same when the three strains of mice are arranged according to their liability to develop pituitary tumours, but the two treatments also appear to need a comparable time for pituitary tumours to develop as well as for them to attain the maximum size that is compatible with life. This is what may be expected if there is a common pathway. Even the observed dissociation between the tumour inducing efficiencies of the two types of hormonal derangements in C_3H_f mice and R-Amsterdam rats, respectively, does not necessary preclude a common pathway. The results could be interpreted to suggest that in most strains of mice a common pituitary tumour induction mechanism can be set in motion by either of the two types of hormonal derangement, but that in C_3H_f mice continuous oestrone administration fails to "turn the switch" that sets the common mechanism in motion and that in rats thyroid hormone deficiency fails to do so.

In this reasoning much importance is given to the "close parallelism" in induction time and growth rate of the pituitary tumours induced by either of the two hormonal imbalances in each of the three strains of mice. A method was needed therefore that would allow statistical analysis of the possible existence of such a parallelism in the growth processes induced by the two types of hormonal derangement. The theory of CLIFTON and MEYER (1956 b, see II. 4. a.) appeared to suggest such an analysis. It was claimed to provide a basis for a theoretical growth curve that parallels closely the observed weights of pituitary tumours induced by oestrogens in rats. The assumptions of CLIFTON and MEYER are that the specific hormonal derangement, i. e. continuous stimulation by oestrogens, induces an enhanced mitotic rate in those pituitary cells that are stimulated by oestrogens and in the progeny of these cells only. This enhanced mitotic activity exceeds the requirements for normal cell replacement and, provided that the mitotic rate is constantly elevated above the normal requirement, an increase in the number of this family of stimulated cells takes place. The increase proceeds according to a geometrical progression. For practical purposes this means that the number of cells of the particular type will double at a constant time interval (t^d), i. e. when the process affects 100 cells of the normal pituitary cell population, the number of this particular type will be 200, t^d days later; 400 another t^d days later, etc. In the rats used by CLIFTON and MEYER this constant time interval appears to be 30 days and the number of cells stimulated to enhanced mitotic activity is stated to be 1% of the normal cell population of the rat pituitary. According to their theory the cell type stimulated by oestrogens is the "prolactin producing" eosinophile cell.

Theoretical growth curves were drawn on the assumptions that all the cells of the pituitary, 30% of the normal cell population, 10%, 3% and 1% respectively are stimulated to enhanced mitotic activity, (see Fig. 1). The calculated pituitary weights were plotted on the vertical axis of a logarithmic scale; the horizontal axis represents the scale on which t^d represents the time necessary for the proliferating cells to double in number. When the theoretical pituitary weights are thus expressed graphically on a semi-logarithmic scale it is obvious that the growth curve will be represented by a *straight line* when all the cells divide; the straight line will depart from the horizontal immediately the cells begin to proliferate and the angle it makes with the horizontal depends only on the scale chosen to plot the time necessary to double the number of participating cells. The theoretical growth curves for the other proportions of dividing cells demonstrate clearly that all the curves will eventually approach a straight line and that the straight part of all these other assumed growth curves will run parallel to the straight line representing the case where all cells proliferate: In other words the angle that is formed by the straight part of the curve is not influenced by the proportion of the

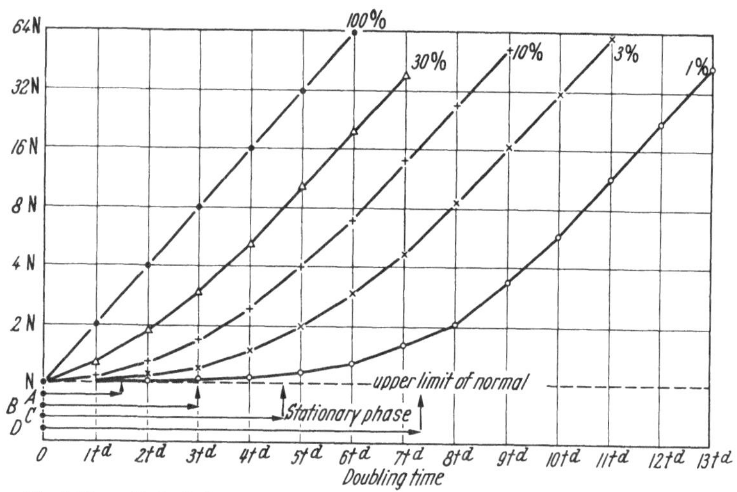

Fig. 1. Theoretical pituitary weight curves: % of normal cell population participating in tumour process

normal pituitary cell population that proliferates; only the duration of the apparent "stationary phase" is influenced.

In Fig. 2 the observed pituitary weights of orchidectomized R-Amsterdam rats, treated with oestrone are plotted in this way. The scale on which the duration of treatment has been plotted on the horizontal axis has been so chosen that the calculated time that is necessary for the pituitaries to double in weight approximates to the t^d scale of Fig. 1 in order to facilitate comparison of the theoretical growth curves and the observed weights. The two graphs demonstrate that the results in the orchidectomized R-Amsterdam rats, are remarkably consistent with the theory of Clifton and Meyer and with their results in Sprague Dawley rats, since there is fair agreement with their conclusions on the percentage of cell of the normal pituitary participating in the process of proliferation as well as on the "doubling time". Adopting their theory that the

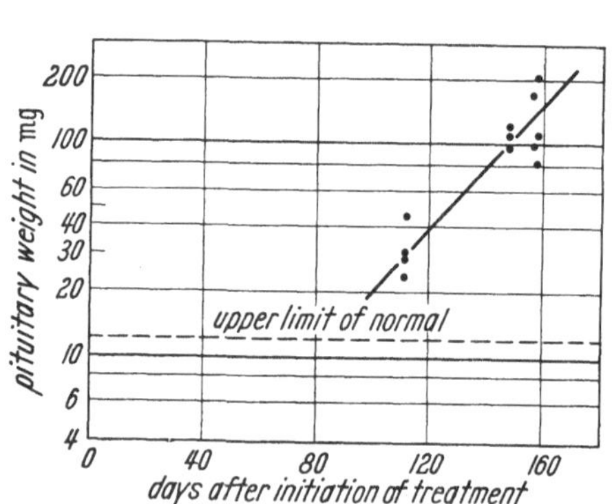

Fig. 2. Pituitary tumours in orchidectomized ♂♂ rats R-Amsterdam by continuous oestrone administration

enhancement of the mitotic rate caused by oestrogens sets in immediately and therefore coincides with the beginning of treatment the results of the present experiment suggest approximately 3% and approximately 20 days respectively, compared to 1% and 30 days in their experiment.

The observed pituitary weights of female strain R-Amsterdam rats, treated with oestrone showed, however, an entirely different growth curve, represented in Fig. 3. Again the time scale has been so chosen as to facilitate comparison with Fig. 1. The growth rate of the tumours in female rats is much slower than in the orchidectomized male rats, the "doubling" times being calculated as approximately 50 days and 20 days respectively. But the most striking difference is the position of the straight part of the growth curve, which suggests that far more than 1% or 3% of the cell population of the normal pituitary must have been engaged in cell proliferation; an estimate that between 10% and 90% of the cell population of the pituitary participated at the beginning of the oestrone treatment would be more consistent. This suggests either that the "prolactin producing" eosinophile cell type make up a much larger percentage of the normal cell population of the pituitary in the female rats than in the male rats, or that the assumption of CLIFTON and MEYER that the beginning of the proliferation process coincides with the beginning of oestrone treatment, is not tenable. It should be pointed out that, if the time of onset of the process of proliferation is unknown it would be very difficult, if not impossible, to do more than estimate the minimum percentage of cells participating in the process. This can be demonstrated by Fig. 1. The theoretical growth curve to which the "stationary phase" D belongs may represent either a process of cell proliferation that begins immediately after the initiation of treatment and that engages only 1% of the population of the pituitary cells, or a process of cell proliferation that eventually engages every cell of the pituitary but which begins only many months after the initiation of treatment. The difference is that in the first case the stationary phase is an apparent one, during which the numerical increase of cells is not reflected appreciably in the weight of the pituitary, whereas in the second case the stationary phase is a true one, during which no numerical increase of cells take place. The duration of the apparent stationary phase therefore is alone relevant to the percentage of cells of the normal population that participate in the process. When the onset of proliferation in relation to the beginning of treatment is unknown, the assumption that they coincide may result in a too low estimate. It will never result in too high an estimate provided that the allowance made for the increase in cell volume, increase in vascularity, etc. has been correct.

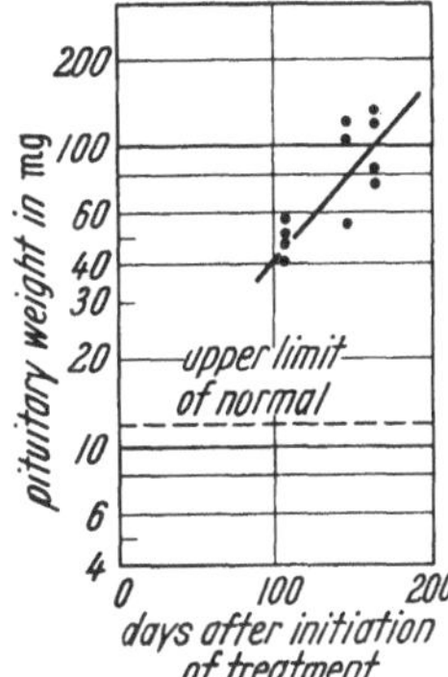

Fig. 3. Pituitary tumours in ♀♀ rats R-Amsterdam by continuous oestrone administration

The pituitary weights observed in orchidectomized male C_{57}Bl mice given 2 mg of oestrone per liter of drinking water are represented in the same way in Fig. 4. The time scale has been so chosen as to facilitate comparison with Fig. 1. Whereas the number of observations on the rat pituitary weights were not sufficiently spread along the time axis to prove or to disprove that the pituitary weight increases exponentially with time as implied by the theory of CLIFTON and MEYER, the C_{57}Bl pituitary weights cluster indeed very well around a straight line, with the possible exception of the "oldest" specimens, thus supporting the above mentioned theory.

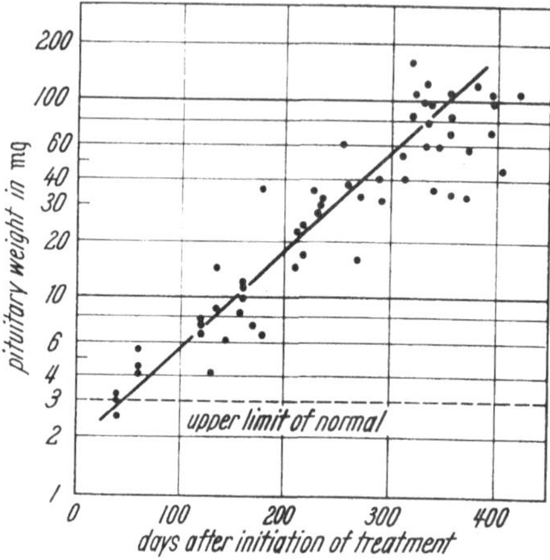

Fig. 4. Pituitary tumours in orchidectomized ♂♂ C_{57}Bl by continuous oestrone administration

The growth rate is comparable to that observed in the female rats, the "doubling time" being approximately 50 days. The position of the straight part of the curve suggests that approximately 30% of the cell population is involved, assuming that the beginning of the proliferation process coincides with the initiation of treatment.

The pituitary weights observed in the C_{57}Bl male, female and spayed female mice suggested that there was no "sex-difference" in the pituitary tumour growth rate. The growth curves of these three groups of C_{57}Bl mice, however, were "shifted slightly to the right" in comparison with the curve found in the orchidectomized males.

Adopting all the assumptions of CLIFTON and MEYER the growth curves in the C_{57}Bl mice, would be interpreted as showing that the "prolactin producing" eosinophile cells make up between 10% and 30% of the normal pituitary cell population. This estimate may be considered in fair agreement with the changes seen in the pituitary of the female mouse during the oestrus cycle. The eosinophile cells make up about 40% of the cells in the pituitary during di-oestrus (VAN EBBENHORST-TENGBERGEN, 1955); from early pro-oestrus to late pro-oestrus this percentage drops to 30%, owing, it is presumed, to the degranulation that is observed in the eosinophile cells. Since the eosinophile cells are also agreed to be the site of growth hormone production and probably also of ACTH (see Table 1; page 10, II. 3. b.) and the release of neither of these two hormones is likely to undergo extreme shifts correlated with the oestrus cycle, the eosinophile cells, which completely degranulate and become fully granulated again in correlation with the oestrus cycle and which make up about 10% of the cells in the normal female pituitary, may be inferred to be the site of production of prolactin in the mouse.

Whereas the growth curve of the oestrone-induced pituitary tumours can be interpreted as being consistent with the proposition that these tumours originate exclusively from the "prolactin producing" cells and thus appear to support the "monomorphous and monohormonal" concept of the experimentally induced pituitary tumours of FURTH (see II. 4. a.), the growth curves (Fig. 6, 8 and 10) of pituitary tumours developing in mice after a thyroid-destructive dose of ^{131}I are an almost decisive rejection of FURTH's view that these tumours originate exclusively from the TSH producing cells, the "thyrotropes". The position of the "straight part of the curve" in regard to the time of administration of the thyroid-destructive dose of radioactive iodine in all these examples indicates that the "radiothyroidectomy"-induced pituitary tumours originate from a family of pituitary cells, which make up between 10% and 30% of the cell population of the normal pituitary; they can not have originated exclusively from a cell type that makes up such a relatively small number as the "thyrotropes" do in the pituitary of a normal mouse. The "thyrotropes" belong to the basophile line of cells and in the mouse pituitary the number of true basophile cells, "deep blue staining, grossly granulated cells", is so small that they have been disregarded in differential counts of pituitary cells in various phases of the oestrus cycle (VAN EBBENHORST-TENGBERGEN, 1955). It would be necessary to count an impracticably large total number of pituitary cells to disclose statistically valid differences in the proportions of basophile cells (VAN EBBENHORST-TENGBERGEN, personal communication). This is in agreement with personal experience with the very sensitive PAS modification of RUYTER (1958, see IV. B.). In the pituitaries of untreated mice of various strains on the normal regimen in the Netherlands Cancer Institute the numbers of PAS-positive cells per section in serial sections of the same pituitary gland range from 0 to 7, so that an estimate that less than 1% of the cells of a normal pituitary of a mouse stain PAS-positive appears to be justified. Since cells containing PAS-positive granules include the FSH- and LH-producing cells besides the TSH producing "thyrotropes", the pituitary tumour growth curves suggest either that undifferentiated cells, which contribute to tumour formation, exist along with the fully differentiated cells and make up about 10% or more of the cell population, or that the concept that the "radiothyroidectomy"-induced pituitary tumour is a „monomorphous mass of TSH secreting cells" must be abandoned in favour of the concept that a tumour consists of more than one type of cell proliferating without limit.

In Fig. 5 to 10 three examples are given to illustrate the striking similarity of the growth curves of pituitary tumours induced by oestrone and by "radiothyroidectomy". (The time scale is the same for all the graphs representing the growth curves in mice). The growth curves of pituitary tumours in male C_{57}Bl mice (5 and 6); in orchidectomized male (C_{57}Bl × DBA_f) F_1 mice (7 and 8) and in female (C_{57}Bl × DBA_f) F_1 mice (9 and 10) induced by oestrone and by "radiothyroidectomy" respectively are represented. Statistical evaluation by analysis of covariance[1] showed that there are no indications whatsoever to conclude that the oestrone growth curve and the "radiothyroidectomy" growth curve are not identical in each pair of comparable groups of mice.

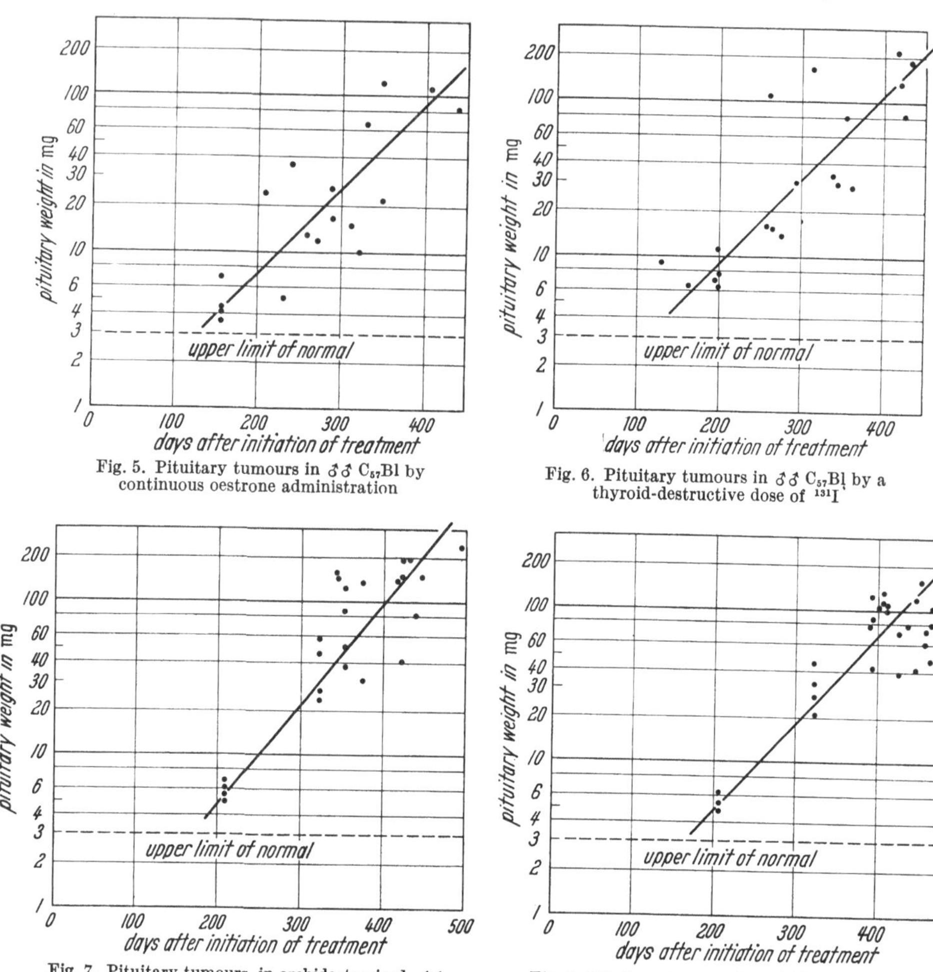

Fig. 5. Pituitary tumours in ♂♂ $C_{57}Bl$ by continuous oestrone administration

Fig. 6. Pituitary tumours in ♂♂ $C_{57}Bl$ by a thyroid-destructive dose of ^{131}I

Fig. 7. Pituitary tumours in orchidectomized ♂♂ $[C_{57}Bl \times DBAf]F_1$ by continuous oestrone administration

Fig. 8. Pituitary tumours in orchidectomized ♂♂ $[C_{57}Bl \times DBAf]F_1$ by a thyroid-destructive dose of ^{131}I

Whereas there was no detectable difference between the growth curves of pituitary tumours induced by the two types of hormonal

[1] Statistical theory gives a method, the so called analysis of covariance (see Dixon and Massey, page 37), to examine whether the straight lines fitted to various groups of observations can be considered as being identical, or parallel, or as differing in slope. The method is based on some assumptions, e. g. that the observations have a normal probability distribution, that they are distributed around a straight line, etc., which have been assumed to hold for the pituitary weight data of the present experiment.

derangement, the difference in slope between the growth curves of the orchidectomized males and the females of the (C_{57}Bl × DBA_f) F_1 hybrids

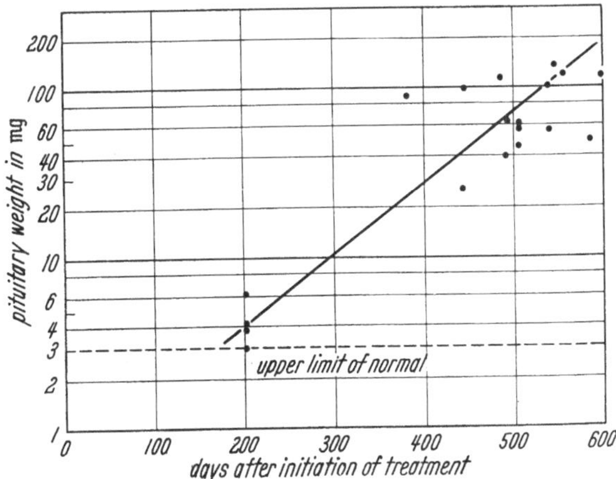

Fig. 9. Pituitary tumours in spayed ♀♀ [C_{57}Bl × DBA_f]F_1 by continuous oestrone administration

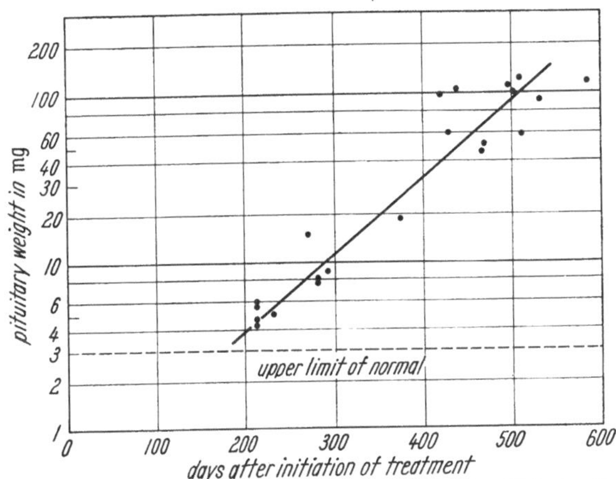

Fig. 10. Pituitary tumours in spayed ♀♀ [C_{57}Bl × DBA_f]F_1 by a thyroid-destructive dose of ^{131}I

was statistically significant at the $p < .01$ level. The observed pituitary weights in the spayed females of this hybrid suggested that castration does not affect the growth curves of the pituitary tumours in females. The results in the (O_{20} × DBA_f) F_1 hybrids suggested also an "identical" growth curve for the oestrone-induced and for the "radiothyroidectomy"-induced pituitary tumours as well as a comparable sex-linked difference in the slope between males and females; the observed pituitary weights in these hybrids were too few in number and were not suitably dispersed along the time axis to calculate a growth curve and statistical confirmation was therefore not possible. As mentioned earlier no indication of such a sex-linked difference in slope was found in the C_{57}Bl strain.

The results of classifying the pituitaries according to weight (Table 3) suggested a genetically determined difference in induction time and rate of growth of pituitary tumours. The growth curves indicate that a major part of the observed "superiority" of the C_{57}Bl mice over the (C_{57}Bl × DBA$_f$) F_1 hybrids may be attributed to this sex-linked difference in the slope of the growth curve in the hybrids; the growth curves of the orchidectomized males of these hybrids does not differ significantly in slope from the growth curves in the C_{57}Bl mice. The results in the (O_{20} × DBA$_f$) F_1 hybrids suggests a "flatter" slope compared to either the C_{57}Bl or the (C_{57}Bl × DBA$_f$) F_1 hybrids but statistical confirmation of this impression was not possible (see above). Data on the pituitary weights in male mice of the WLL$_{e/f}$ strain which were suitably dispersed along the time axis were available, for calculating the growth curve represented in Fig. 11. The slope of this curve is also much "flatter" than the one found for the oestrone-induced pituitary tumours in the C_{57}Bl male, the difference in slope being statistically significant.

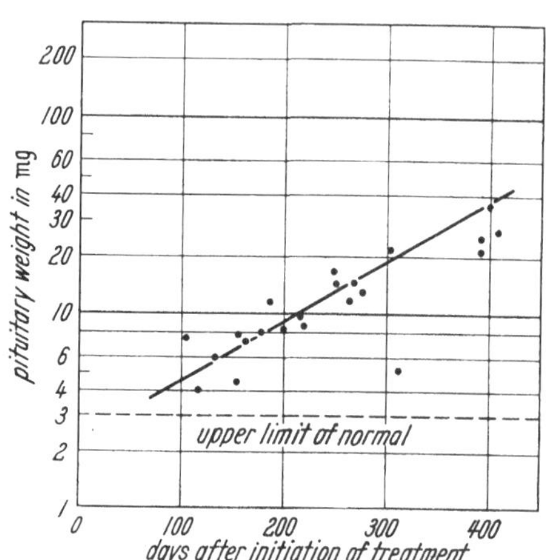

Fig. 11. Pituitary tumours in ♂♂ WLL$_{f/e}$ by continuous oestrone administration

Except for the growth curve in orchidectomized male rats, all growth curves thus far discussed, including those in female rats as well as in mice suggest that a much greater percentage of the normal population of pituitary cells take part in the unrestrained proliferation than Clifton and Meyer proposed for the rat pituitary stimulated by oestrogens. It has been mentioned that the differences in growth curves found in the present experiment between orchidectomized male rats (1. b.) and female rats (1. c.) were two-fold; a difference in growth rate between males and females comparable to that found in the two hybrid-strains in the mouse experiments, and a difference in position of the "straight part of the curve" in regard to the initiation of treatment. Two hypotheses were considered possible. Either the normal male pituitary in comparison with the female pituitary contains only few of the prolactin producing eosinophile cells, which are presumed to respond to oestrone by enhanced mitotic activity or the orchidectomized male rat is resistant to oestrone stimulation for a considerable time so that there is a *true* stationary phase. The pituitary cells start to proliferate only when this "resistance" is broken down. Since a difference in the percentage of "prolactin producing" eosinophile cells cannot be excluded a priori, both hypotheses explain equally well the observed difference in position of the straight part of the growth curve. In the (C_{57}Bl × DBA$_f$) F_1 hybrids, however, a similar difference in the position of the straight parts of the pituitary tumour growth curves was found between males and orchidectomized males (Fig. 12.). Because orchidectomy was carried out on the same day as the oestrone regimen was started, a difference in the percentages of the different pituitary cell types at the beginning of treatment seems out of the question. It appears more probable that a *true* stationary phase rather than a difference in number of "oestrone-sensitive" cells is responsible for the difference in position of the straight

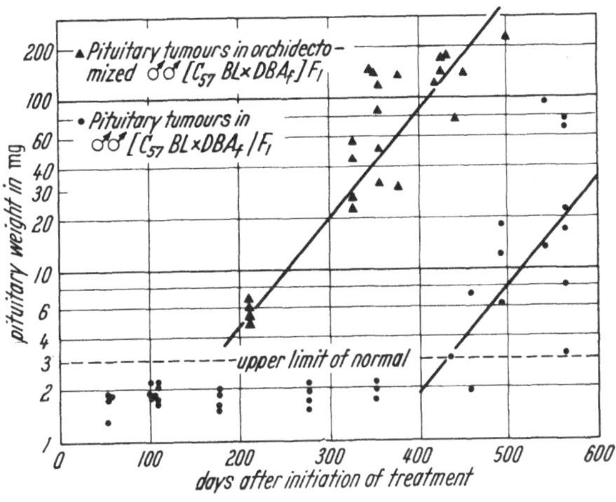

Fig. 12. Comparison of weight curves of pituitary tumours in intact and orchidectomized ♂♂ [C_{57}Bl × DBAf]F_1 by continuous oestrone administration

part of the growth curve in the male. Therefore the second alternative that a "resistance" to hyperoestrogenization may exist seems more probable. In agreement with this proposition is the finding that once proliferation begins in the intact males the observed pituitary weights are suggestive of a growth rate, which is represented by the slope of the straight part of the curve, corresponding with that found in orchidectomized males.

These data suggest that; a) the type of hormonal derangement does not influence the rate of growth of pituitary tumours, whereas b) the sex of the animal, as well as c) the genetic constitution may do so. They are strongly suggestive therefore of the existence of a *common pathway* in the induction mechanism after either of the two types of hormonal derangement. Moreover the data suggest that pituitary tumour formation is an "all-or-none phenomenon", which can be provoked by various hormonal derangements, rather than a graded response that is more or less quantitatively related to the strength of the stimulus employed. Otherwise it is difficult to understand how oestrone excess and thyroid hormone deprivation both result in an "identical" growth rate of the induced pituitary tumours. Even if the type of the proliferating cells is ignored, the finding of an identical pair of growth curves implies that by coincidence the dose of oestrone used in this experiment stimulated the mitotic activity of the pituitary cells to exactly the same degree as does thyroid hormone deficiency, which acts by removing an inhibition (see II. 4.). The finding that in all groups of mice in which the data were suitable for statistical analysis, the growth rates of the pituitary tumours induced by the two hormonal derangements were "identical", strongly suggests that this correspondence in growth rates is not fortuitous.

The recently reported finding that normal pituitaries isografted subcutaneously may develop at the site of implantation into chromophobic pituitary tumours which may reach a weight of 500 mg (MÜHLBOCK and BOOT, 1959), suggests that the hypothalamus normally exerts a regulatory action on mitotic activity in the pituitary. The following working hypothesis is proposed: The mitotic rate of the pituitary cells is under control of a regulating centre in the hypothalamus, which normally adjusts it to physiological requirements. When the pituitary "escapes" from this control, either by being isografted at a site away from the hypothalamus, or when the hypothalamic centre is "overwhelmed" by oestrogen excess or by thyroid hormone deficiency, a pituitary tumour develops. Apparently in the C_3H-strain of mice the hypothalamus is more resistant to oestrone excess and remains capable of exerting its regulatory action on mitotic activity, whereas the rat hypothalamus appears to be resistant to thyroid hormone deficiency.

As to the type of pituitary cells that develop into pituitary tumours, the "identical" growth curves suggest that one and the same cell type, (for instance the "amphophile cell", if it is conceived as the multipotent, undifferentiated cell existing along with the fully differentiated ones in the normal pituitary), is stimulated to an enhanced mitotic activity by both types of hormonal derangement. However, the possibility should be emphasized that the various "fully differentiated" cell types in the pituitary, may all have inherited the same "growth potential", since they all stem from the "pituitary mother cell".

The possibility cannot be excluded that the *oestrone-induced* pituitary tumours originate exclusively from the fully differentiated "prolactin producing eosinophile" cells and thus the growth curve may be interpreted as consistent with a monomorphous monohormonal concept for this type of tumour. For the *"radiothyroidectomy"-induced* pituitary tumours, however, the growth curves are not consistent with the view that these pituitary tumours originate exclusively from the fully differentiated, "TSH producing, PAS-positive basophile" cells.

When the pituitary tumour that is induced by thyroid hormone deficiency is considered as a "monomorphous, monohormonal" tumour, either a considerable number of undifferentiated cells must be presumed to exist along with the fully differentiated ones in the normal pituitary and these cells must contribute to the tumour development and differentiate into TSH-producing cells during the process, or one or more of the "fully differentiated" cell types must change into TSH-producing tumour cells. If the different functional cell types are viewed as irreversibly differentiated cells, the concept of the pituitary as "a mosaic of different functional cell types, independently regulating specific functions" is not consistent with the present findings for the "radiothyroidectomy"-induced pituitary tumours.

The close correspondence in growth rates found between the oestrone-induced and the "radiothyroidectomy"-induced pituitary tumours thus poses the question whether these tumours are morphologically and functionally different.

IV. Morphological characteristics of experimental pituitary tumours of mice of different inbred strains

This chapter deals with the morphology of pituitary tumours induced in mice either by continuous oestrone administration or by thyroid hormone deficiency.

It has been postulated that these two types of tumours originate from the "prolactin producing eosinophile cells" and from the "TSH producing basophile cells" respectively (see II. 4. a.). The close correspondence in growth rate of these tumours (see discussion and conclusions III.) appeared to be more consistent with the view that both types of tumours originate from the same pituitary cell type (II. 4. b.). A comparison of the morphological aspects is desirable since it may provide evidence of decisive value for the disputed question of the origin of the tumours in question and of pituitary tumours in general.

The first part of this chapter evaluates the modified Mallory tri-chrome stain commonly used in this laboratory for the differentiation of the two types of pituitary tumours mentioned and the second part deals with the PAS reaction (*p*eriodic-*a*cid *S*chiff reaction).

A. Comparison of the morphology of oestrone-induced and "radiothyroidectomy"-induced pituitary tumours employing a tri-chrome stain

The object of this investigation was to ascertain whether the modified Mallory tri-chrome stain commonly used in this laboratory would suffice to differentiate between the two types of pituitary tumours. The connotation of differently induced pituitary tumours in mice as "thyrotropic", "mammotropic", etc. suggests that such tumours differ morphologically as clearly from each other as the basophilic, rather large and angularly outlined "thyrotropic cell" differs from the eosinophilic, much smaller and round to ovally shaped "mammotropic cell", etc. However, in the mouse pituitary even the classification into the customary three cell types (eosinophilic, basophilic and chromophobic) is difficult, since the non-acidophilic cell types appear hard to define (van Ebbenhorst-Tengbergen, 1955). Moreover in hypertrophic pituitaries even in the rat, where the specific cell types seem to be more distinct, the changes induced in the stimulated cells tend to obscure the initially distinct morphological characteristics. Loss of the specific staining properties occurs when the cells degranulate, differences in cell size between the eosinophilic cells, basophilic cells and chromophobic cells tend to be leveled out as the cells hypertrophy; and the specific types of Golgi apparatus, which appear not to be recognizable in many other species (PEARSE, 1952 b), are replaced by a hypertrophic Golgi apparatus, which is of similar appearance in acidophile cells and basophile cells (SEVERINGHAUS, 1933, 1937; WOLFE, 1949).

1. Material and methods

Pituitary adenomata from $C_{57}Bl$, ($O_{20} \times DBA_f$) F_1 and ($C_{57}Bl \times DBA_f$) F_1 mice, orchidectomized males, intact males, spayed females and intact females were included into this investigation. The pituitary tumours had developed, either after continuous oestrogen treatment, started at the age of six to eleven weeks and continued throughout life, or after destruction of the thyroid gland by an adequate dose of radioactive iodine administered at the age of six to eleven weeks. The material covered serial sections (1 out of five) of 178 pathological mouse pituitaries. For fixation and staining, the modified Zenker-formol and the modified Mallory trichrome technique as described by VAN EBBENHORST-TENGBERGEN (1955) was used.

After a preliminary survey, eight different morphological criteria were adopted. Each criterion gave two, three or four possibilities for classification. It was proposed that all sections should be classified for each of the criteria by three different investigators working independently. The classification was made without knowledge of the treatment that had elicited the tumour.

The objectivity of the different criteria was evaluated by submitting the independently obtained classifications to a statistical analysis (VAN EEDEN, 1953).

The scatter of the different classifications for each of the eight criteria in the oestrone- and in the "radiothyroidectomy"-groups as well as in comparable pairs of sub-groups (for strain- and sex-differences) were then compared and the statistical significance of any difference was evaluated according to the method described by VAN EEDEN and RUMKE (1958).

The criteria adopted as promising to be of most value in differentiating between the two treatment groups were:

1. Extreme polymorphism of the nuclei or polymorphism to a lesser degree, classified respectively as "positive" or "negative".

2. Extreme prominence of the nucleoli, prominence of the nucleoli or no prominence of the nucleoli in the majority of cells.

3. "Presence" or "absence" of chromatin in the nucleus in the majority of cells.

4. Presence or absence of vacuoles in the nucleus in one or more cells per section.

5. Colour taken by the majority of pituitary cells: blue, violet or red.

6. Presence or absence of "blood filled tissue clefts" in the pituitary sections.

7. Size of the majority of cells: large, medium or small.

8. Cell shape[1], classified as "round", "indefinite", "angular" or "stellate".

During oral consultations the first four criteria were proposed by Miss Cardauns of the Max-Planck-Institut für Hirnforschung (Köln), the two next criteria by Miss W.J.P.R. VAN EBBENHORST-TENGBERGEN, of the Netherlands Cancer Institute, the last two criteria were later included on the advice of Dr. F. BIELSCHOWSKY, (Dunedin, New Zealand).

2. Results

The results of the statistical analysis as to whether the agreement in classification by the three independent investigators could have been due to chance are given in Table 8. As can be seen the last seven criteria definitely substantiated the claim of objectivity, while even the first criterion may have had some objective value as the two most experienced workers in pituitary histology (Miss C. and Miss T.) obtained rather good agreement.

Table 8. *Correlation of the classification results obtained by the three participators*

Criterion	p values[2] obtained between		
	C and T or[3] O and T	C and K or[3] O and K	T and K
iso- or polymorphy of the nucleus	$p = 0.0019$	$p = 0.166$	$p = 0.462$
prominence of the nucleolus	$p < 0.0004$	$p < 0.0004$	$p < 0.0004$
chromatin content of the nucleus	$p < 0.0004$	$p < 0.0004$	$p < 0.0004$
presence of vacuoles in the nucleus	$p = 0.0007$	$p = 0.0073$	$p < 0.0004$
colour of the cells	$p < 0.0004$	$p < 0.0004$	$p < 0.0004$
"bloodfilled tissueclefts"	$p < 0.0004$	$p < 0.0004$	$p < 0.0004$
size of the cells	$p < 0.0004$	$p < 0.0004$	$p < 0.0004$
shape of the cells	$p < 0.0004$	$p < 0.0004$	$p < 0.0004$

[1] The criterion of cell shape was adopted on the basis of the difference between the round or oval (eosinophilic) "mammotrope" and the angular outlines of the (basophilic) "thyrotrope". The obvious difficulty was that even in the normal pituitary the eosinophile cell is often more or less angular due to compression by neighbouring cells. As this would classify all pituitary tumours as "angular", the cell-shape was considered rather to reflect "cell turgor" and shapes regarded to be consistent with good "cell turgor" were classified as "round", whereas cells showing shapes more consistent with lack of "cell turgor" were classified to be "angular". Therefore special attention was paid to areas where cells were not compressed by other cells on all sides, such as in areas bordering bloodsinuses, etc. The extreme case of "lack of cell turgor" was recognized when a cell compressed by its neighbouring cells showed a strand of protoplasma between two other cells as long as the diameter of these cells or more. Such cells were classified as "stellate". This classification had the drawback that the shape of only a few cells in one or two areas often decided the evaluation of the whole pituitary gland.

[2] The probability (p) that the correlation obtained by two independent participators had been due to chance was calculated according to the method described by VAN EEDEN (1953).

[3] Whereas T and K participated in the classification of all the eight criteria, Miss C participated only in the first six criteria, the classification of the last two criteria were done by Mr. Oei, O.L.

The distribution of the classifications for each of the eight criteria over the oestrone- and over the "radiothyroidectomy"-group were as follows:

Polymorphism of the nucleus proved to be of no value for differentiating the two treatment groups, as 70.4% in the oestrone group against 74.5% in the "radiothyroidectomy" group was so classified. The difference had no statistical significance ($p = 0.131$).

Prominence of the nucleolus: the difference in distribution between the two treatment groups was too small to have any practical value. Oestrone group: 16.1% extreme prominence, 35.7% prominence and 48.2% no prominence of the nucleolus, against the "thyroidectomy" group: 15.7% extreme prominence, 42.3% prominence and 42.0% no prominence of the nucleoli. The difference had no statistical value ($p = 0.0628$).

A pecularity was that there appeared to be a statistically significant strain difference in the reaction to "radiothyroidectomy". The Bd_fF_1 showed more and/or more definite prominence of the nucleoli:

	++	+	–		
$C_{57}Bl$	8.0%	34.7%	57.3%		
				$p < 0.01$	
Bd_fF_1	29.6 %	42.5%	27.8%		$p = 0.10$
				$p = 0.03$	
Od_fF_1	2.8%	64.4%	32.8%		

Chromatin content of the nucleus: the difference between the distributions in the two treatment groups for this criterion was small and statistically not significant for all strains taken together. In the oestrone group 43.4% of the sections were classified as positive against 40.0% positives in the "thyroidectomy" group ($p = 0.5824$). However, when the Bd_fF_1 were considered separately 66.7% were classified in the oestrone group as positive against 40.7% in the "thyreoidectomy" group, the difference being statistically significant ($p = 0.02$). This was due to the tendency of the Bd_fF_1 to show more chromatin in the nucleus after oestrone treatment than the Od_fF_1 (statistically not significant or than the $C_{57}Bl$ statistically significant).

Presence of vacuoles in the nucleus: was encountered more in the "radiothyroidectomy" group than in the oestrone group in all three strains of mice. This difference was very distinct in the Od_fF_1 and much less so in the two other strains (not statistically significant, in the case of $C_{57}Bl$: $p = 0.13$, or Bd_fF_1: $p = 0.12$). However for all strains taken together the difference was statistically significant, in the oestrone group 23.8% being classified as positive against 46.3% positives in the "radiothyroidectomy" group ($p < 0.0004$). For the Od_fF_1 pituitaries the corresponding percentages were respectively 9.5% and 66.7% ($p = 0.0058$), so it was only for the differentiation of pituitary tumours in this hybrid that the criterium promised to be of some practical value.

Colour taken by the majority of cells after staining with the Mallory tri-chrome modification used showed definitely more blue in the "radiothyroidectomy" group, probably reflecting a greater RNA-content of the cytoplasm after this type of hormonal imbalance:

	blue	lilac	red	
oestrone group	19.0%	50.0%	31.0%	$p < 0.0004$
"radiothyroidectomy" group	53.5%	36.5%	11.0%	

The females $BdfF_1$ were the only exception to this general tendency showing no difference between the two treatment groups, owing to a definite sex difference in this hybrid mouse after "radiothyroidectomy". Castration abolished this sex difference.

After "radiothyroidectomy":	blue	lilac	red	
male $BdfF_1$	26.6%	60.0%	13.4%	$p = 0.0427$
female $BdfF_1$	6.6%	53.4%	40.0%	
castrated male $BdfF_1$	66.7%	30.3%	3.0%	$p > 0.90$
spayed female $BdfF_1$	66.3%	36.7%	0.0%	

(p value for the difference between female and spayed female: $p = 0.008$)

"*Bloodfilled tissue clefts*" occurred in 77.4% of the oestrone sections against 55.7% of the "radiothyroidectomy" group, the difference being statistically significant ($p < 0.0004$).

Size of the majority of cells tended to differ between the oestrone and the "radiothyroidectomy" groups. The percentage distribution over the three adopted classifications was:

	large	*medium*	*small*	
oestrone group	14.2%	42.9%	42.9%	$p < 0.0004$
"radiothyroidectomy" group	57.7%	37.6%	4.7%	

Shape of the cells: the difference between the oestrone and the "radiothyroidectomy" groups in the distributions over the four classifications adopted for this criterion was quite distinct:

	round	indefinite	angular	stellate	
oestrone	51.8%	40.1%	7.1%	0.0%	$p < 0.0004$
"radiothyroidectomy"	0.0%	22.4%	70.6%	7.0%	

3. Discussion

The Mallory tri-chrome staining technique does not give satisfactory results when applied to the differently induced pituitary tumours in mice, as on a strictly descriptive basis all these tumours should be classified as "chromophobic"; the application of terms such as "degranulated basophiles" or "degranulated acidophiles' only introduces the authors opinion of the origin of the tumour cells into his description of the different pituitary tumours.

Within the limits of what could be expected from our material stained with the Mallory tri-chrome technique, the method of approach may be stated to have fulfilled the objectives. Seven out of the eight criteria used in this investigation appeared to be sufficiently objective and distinct for even less experienced participators to obtain good agreement in assessment.

The criterion of more or less pronounced polymorphism of the nucleus appeared to be the most difficult to apply. But even when only the satisfactorily correlated classifications of the two experienced observers were taken into account (as has been done) the difference between the two treatment groups was very small and had statistically no significance.

From the seven remaining criteria four may possibly be more or less directly related to the metabolic activity of the pituitary cells:

Loss of chromatin, when the nuclei in the majority of cells are large and vesicular and prominence of the nucleoli have been thought to signify enhanced protein synthesis (WOLFE, 1949; BURT, c.s. 1954).

Ribonucleic acid (RNA) is strongly basophilic and the affinity for the basic dyes as reflected in the blue or lilac colour of the cytoplasm which almost completely disappears after treatment with rubonuclease, may therefore be another indication of the protein metabolism of these cells.

The finding of blood" filled tissue clefts" could be interpreted as reflecting an increased blood supply of the pituitary gland, which would also be consistent with an increased metabolic activity.

The classifications by these four criteria were consistent with an enhanced (protein) metabolism in more than half of the sections (NB not necessarily the same sections for each of the four criteria) in both treatment groups, indicating that the difference between the two groups of pituitary tumours as to their physiological activities — for which the criteria could have been parameters — was not great. A pecularity was that "blood filled tissue clefts" were encountered more often in the oestrone group, whereas more blue cytoplasm as well as loss of chromatin in the nuclei was more often encountered in the "thyroidectomy" group (the differences being statistically significant); prominence of the nucleoli was encountered about equally often in the two treatment groups.

The significance of the vacuoles in the nucleus is not clear. At first they were thought to be enormously enlarged nucleoli, but no correlation between their occurrence and the classification results for the "prominence of the nucleoli" criterion was found. It was interesting that in the Od_fF_1 mice the difference in occurrence of vacuoles in the nucleus was so distinct that this criterion came near to having an absolute value for the differentiation of the type of tumour in this hybrid.

The last two criteria gave statistically significant and quite distinct differences in all subgroups between oestrone- and "radiothyroidectomy"-induced pituitary tumours. As these criteria had been based on two morphological differences between the "thyrotrope" and the "mammotrope" of the normal mouse pituitary, the result could be presumed to fit the concept that the tumours are "thyrotropic" and "mammotropic" and are derived from the two distinct cell types of the normal pituitary gland. However, when it is considered that especially in judging the shape of the cells, the ultimate classification of a pituitary often depended on the shape of only a few cells in one or two areas of the gland, it will be clear that for these criteria too, the differences between the two treatment groups were more of a quantitative than of a qualitative nature.

Seven out of the eight criteria investigated could be correlated with the strain, the sex, or with the treatment of the mouse bearing the tumour or a combination of these. For the differentiation between pituitary tumours induced by the two different hormonal imbalances none of the criteria had an absolute value. The best that may be expected when a Mallory tri-chrome staining technique is employed for the differentiation is a rather good guess if one makes use of the last six criteria.

Both types of hormonal imbalance result in "chromophobic" tumours of the pituitary, as their cells are devoid of granules staining specifically by the trichrome technique. Since the term "chromophobic pituitary adenoma" appears to have acquired the connotation of physiological inactivity (Burt, et al., 1954), it should be pointed out that in both types of tumours morphological characteristics have been found suggestive of an enhanced cellular activity of a possibly endocrine nature.

B. Differentiation of the two types of pituitary tumours by the PAS-reaction

Since the oestrone-induced and the "radiothyroidectomy"-induced pituitary tumours have been presumed to secrete prolactin and TSH respectively (see II. 4. a.) and since the last mentioned hormone is a glyco-protein, whereas the first is not, a differentiation by one of the histochemical reactions for glyco-proteins is suggested.

All pituitary hormones are of protein nature, but only three of them, namely LH (luteinizing hormone); FSH (follicle stimulating hormone) and TSH, are glyco-proteins. It appears that in the normal pituitary the glyco-protein hormones are concentrated in some cells in sufficient amounts to be detectable by the PAS reaction; in the normal pituitary three types of PAS-positive cells have been recognized (see Table 1; II, 3. b.). In the rat pituitary Purves and Griesbach designate them as the "thyrotrophs" the "FSH-gonadotrophs" and the "LH-gonadotrophs" (1957 b), and Halmi (1952, a and b) designates the TSH producing cell as the "beta-cell" and the gonadotrophin producing cell as the "delta-cell". Halmi and Gude (1954) claim that in the normal mouse pituitary "beta"- and "delta-cells" can also be recognized and are of similar appearance as in the rat. They state that the "beta"- and "delta" cells together make up less than 10% of the cell population in the normal mouse pituitary. Whereas the PAS reaction apparently is sufficiently sensitive to detect the amount of TSH that is concentrated in the few "beta-cells or" "thyrotropes" of the normal mouse pituitary it fails to do so in the "highly secreting tumourous "thyrotropes" (FURTH and CLIFTON, 1958). The failure to identify the tumour cells as "thyrotropes" on the basis of known histochemical reactions (FURTH and CLIFTON, 1958) is consistent with the concept of FURTH et al. that the "radiothyroidectomy"-induced pituitary tumours are a "monomorphous mass of secreting thyrotropes", since the reported data on the TSH-content of these tumours suggest that the glycoprotein hormone concentration in tumour cells may be too low to be detectable. BATES, ANDERSON and FURTH (1957) reported that the TSH-assays indicated the presence of the same amount of TSH per unit weight in primary pituitary tumours as in normal pituitaries of mice. The tumours reported were assayed for their TSH content 12 months after the administration of a thyroid-destructive dose of radioactive iodine and had attained weights ranging from 20 mg to 90 mg. A simple calculation shows that the amount of glyco-protein hormone per TSH producing cell in tumours of these sizes is but a fraction of the amount per TSH producing cell of the normal mouse pituitary, since the "thyrotropes" may be presumed to make up the majority of the cells in the tumour (more than 90%), whereas the "thyrotropes" together with the "gonadotropes" have been stated to make up less than 10% of the cells in the pituitary of a normal mouse.

Employing the TSH-assay technique elaborated at the Netherland's Cancer Institute (see V. a.), it was found that the amount of TSH in pituitary tumours, which had attained a mean weight of 30.2 mg 11 month after the administration of a thyroid-destructive dose of radioactive iodine, was more than 1000-fold that of pituitaries of untreated mice of the same strain and age. Since this was a more than fourty-fold increase per unit weight over the normal pituitary, the amount of glyco-protein hormone per cell must have decreased only a little if at all. Thus the chance of obtaining histochemically a positive reaction with the PAS technique appeared to depend on improving the sensitivity of the reaction. The report of a modification of the PAS reaction by RUYTER (1958, a and b), which is claimed to be more sensitive than the usual procedures, suggested the use of this modified PAS reaction.

1. Material and methods

After fixation in Zenker-formol or in Gendre, paraffin sections of pituitary tumours were prepared at 4 micra thickness.

Solutions used for the PAS reaction:

$^1/_2$% periodic acid (made from 50% pro-analyse solution, British Drug House).

Ruyter's modification of the *Schiff* solution:

100 mil. of a $^1/_2$% solution of basic fuchsin is prepared in the usual way, kept overnight at room temperature and is then filtered. To 90 mil. of this solution, 10 mil. of a 20% solution of $K_2S_2O_5$ is added, stirring gently. When the solution is decolourized, it is ready for use. If necessary, activated charcoal may be used. It was found, hewever, that some

batches of activated charcoal can remove the fuchsin nearly quantitatively from the solution.

PAS reaction, technique:

1. Deparaffinize and hydrate as usual.
2. Oxidize in $^1/_2$% periodic acid during 5 min (room temperature).
3. Wash in running tapwater for 3 min.
4. Immerse for $1^1/_2$ to 2 hrs in the modified Schiff-solution.
5. Wash in running tapwater for 5 min.
6. Bring to hydrochloric acid alcohol solution (9 parts of alc 96%, 1 part of 1 n HCl).
7. Counterstain nuclei by haematoxylin or counterstain nuclei, cytoplasm and cytoplasmatic granules by the Mallory trichrome method.

The following procedures to ascertain the nature of the PAS reaction and of the PAS-positive material have been employed:

Prevention of the PAS reaction by acetylation (GERSH), for which the double procedure proposed by McMANUS and CASON, as described by PEARSE (1954) has been followed.

Immersion of the sections for 2 hrs in a $^1/_2$% solution of $K_2S_2O_5$ between the periodic acid step and the sulphite-fuchsin step.

Extraction in boiling chloroform/methanol for 4 hrs, using a reflux condenser over a flask heated in a water bath.

Incubation of the sections at 37° C, immersed in diastase in distilled water for 2 hrs prior to staining.

2. Results

The modification of the PAS technique proposed by RUYTER (1958, a and b), gives a clear cut differentiation between the two types of pituitary tumours (Fig. 14 and 15). The PAS reaction correlates with the TSH-assay results: In the oestrone-induced pituitary tumours of the $(C_{57}Bl \times C_3H_f)F_1$ mice no PAS-positive material could be demonstrated in the pituitary cells and the TSH-assay had proved that the TSH content of the whole tumour was less than in a normal pituitary of an untreated mouse, whereas in "radiothyroidectomy"-induced pituitary tumours of all strains of mice studied thus far a great number of cells contained PAS-positive material. After Zenker-formol fixation the distribution of the PAS-positive material appeared rather blurred, whereas after fixation in *Gendre* the majority of cells show the PAS-positive material in distinct granules. In some cells these granules are so fine and numerous that they appear like "dust".

The PAS reaction becomes negative after acetylation and also no PAS-positive reaction occurs in any of the pituitary cells after immersion in $K_2S_2O_5$-solution. The PAS-positive material is not extracted by boiling chloroform/methanol, and not destroyed by incubation in a diastase solution at 37° C.

3. Discussion

Hormone assays using the prostate weight of hypophysectomized, weanling male rats as criterion indicated that after "radiothyroidectomy" the LH-content of mouse pituitaries is not increased and probably slightly decreased as compared with pituitaries of untreated control mice (unpublished results, J. TUYNMAN, Netherland's Cancer Institute). The testis weights of the hypophysectomized mice used for the TSH-assay

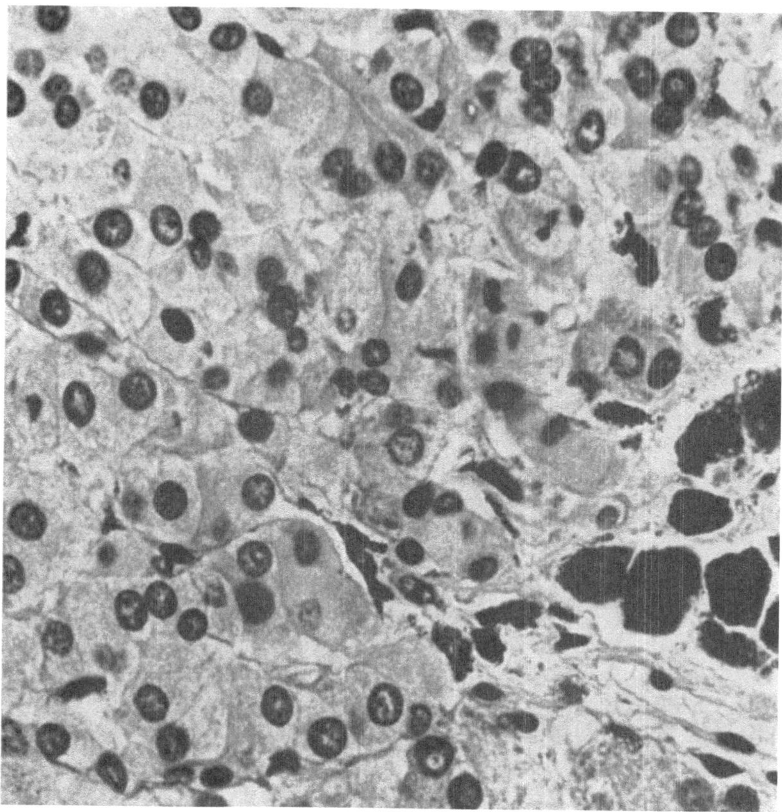

Fig. 13. Pituitary tumour in ♂ C_{57}Bl. (M 132221) 11 months after injection of 200 μC ^{131}I: 4 mμ section stained with the usual PAS procedure. Attention is drawn to the macrophages in the left part of the microphoto: the intensely PAS-positive reaction is due to material of probably lipoid nature in the macrophages, in contrast the pituitary cells do not contain any material that gives a positive reaction with the PAS procedure. (Total enlargement: 800 ×; obj. 40 ×.)

suggested that the FSH-content of the "radiothyroidectomy"-induced pituitary tumours were in the same range as the oestrone-induced pituitary tumours and less than in the pituitaries of the untreated controls, whereas the ^{131}I uptake in the thyroids indicated an enormously increased TSH-content in the "radiothyroidectomy"-induced pituitaries. The histochemical findings in these tumours are consistent with the proposition that the PAS-positive material, which is confined to the intra-cellular granules, represents the thyroid stimulating hormone (TSH) itself or its prescursor.

Ruyter (1958, b) used the number of PAS-positive lymphocytes in air-dried films of human blood as a quantitative criterion for the intensity of the PAS reaction and he reported findings suggestive of an "inhibition" of the PAS reaction by the rinse with sulphite between the periodic acid

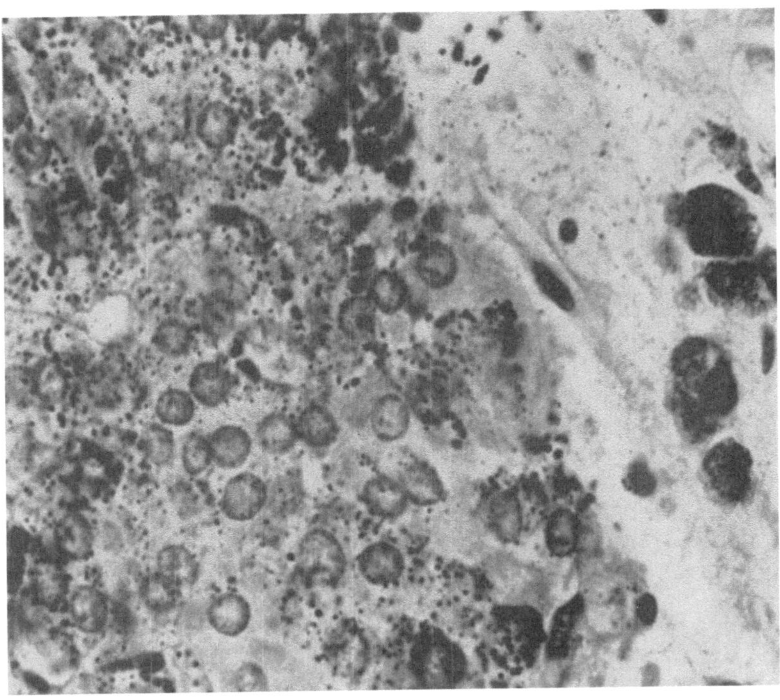

Fig. 14. Pituitary tumour in ♂ C_{57}Bl. (M 132221) 11 months after injection of 200 μC ^{131}I: 4 mμ section stained with Ruyter modification of the PAS procedure; not more than 10 sections apart from the one represented in Fig. 13, approximately the same region is shown in both microphoto's. Compare the intensity of the PAS-positive reaction in the macrophages (in the left part of Fig. 13 and 14): The PAS-positive material in these macrophages has been stained to a comparable intensity by both PAS procedures. With the modified procedure, however, the pituitary cells are shown to contain an abundance of PAS-positive granules. (Total enlargement: 800 ×; obj. 40 ×)

step and the sulphite-fuchsin step (Hotchkiss-technique), since the "blockade" by sulphite of the aldehyde groups that are responsible for the PAS reaction could be decreased by prolonging the immersion time in the sulphite-fuchsin solution. Since even a 24 hrs immersion in the sulphite-fuchsin solution (Ruyter's modification) had no effect on the pituitary sections when immersion in sulphite was interposed between the periodic acid and the sulphite-fuchsin it may be presumed that the "sulphite blockade" of the aldehyde groups of the PAS-positive material in the pituitary tumour cells occurs very easily. The acidity of the medium in the usual Schiff's solutions probably favours the sulphite sufficiently in this "competition" for the aldehyde groups between sulphite and fuchsin to prevent a reaction of the fuchsin with the aldehyde groups. Thus the failure of the usual PAS procedures to stain the granules in the "radiothyroidectomy"-induced pituitary tumours (compare Fig. 13 and 14) may be accounted for.

The seemingly contradictory findings of a close correspondence in growth rate of pituitary tumours induced by oestrone and those induced

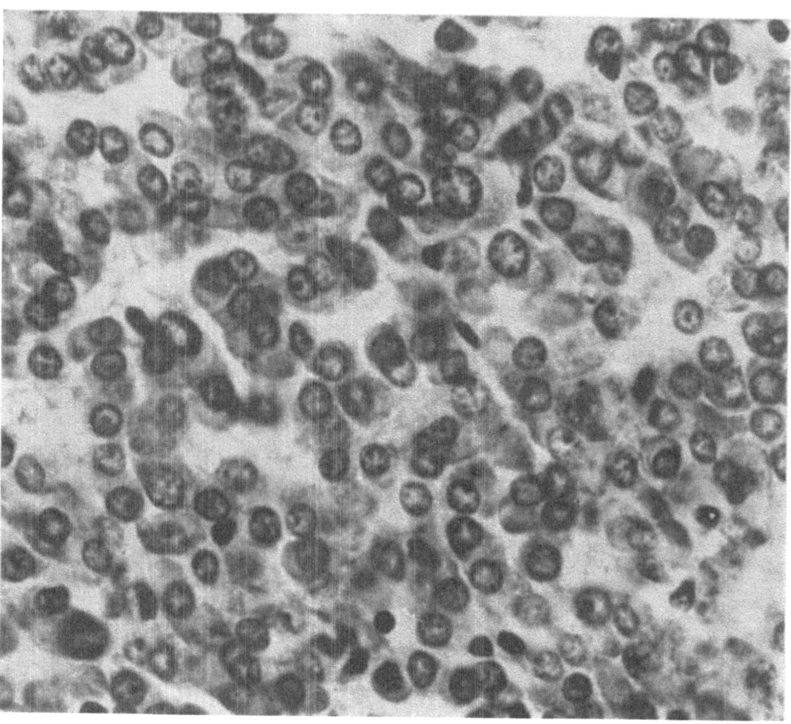

Fig. 15. Pituitary tumours in ♂ ($C_{57}Bl \times C_3Hf$) F_1 (M 118694) 12 months after starting the oestrone in drinking water regimen (2 mg/l tapwater). 4 mμ section stained with the RUYTER modification of the PAS procedure. The oestrone-induced pituitary tumours in this hybrid contain very little TSH. Even after staining with the very sensitive modification (RUYTER) of the PAS-procedure no PAS-positive material was found in the cells of these pituitary tumours. (Total enlargement: 800 ×; obj. 40 ×)

by "radiothyroidectomy" and the clear cut differentiation between the two types of tumours obtained with the modified PAS reaction, suggest the following two alternative working hypotheses for further investigations on the origin and nature of pituitary tumours: firstly, in the normal pituitary of the mouse a relatively large percentage of undifferentiated cells must be presumed to exist along with the fully differentiated ones; these undifferentiated cells proliferate and develop into tumours and differentiate into the specific cell type in accordance with the demand imposed by the hormonal imbalance, or, secondly, the differentiation into various specific cell types in the normal pituitary of the mouse is not an irreversible one, i.e. the various morphologically and functionally distinct cell types of the pituitary may change one into another. Thus pituitary cells of all types may contribute to the development of a "monomorphous" pituitary tumour, which consists exclusively of the specific cell type that can fullfil the demand imposed by the hormonal imbalance.

V. The thyroid stimulating hormone (TSH) content of experimentally induced pituitary tumours in mice

The study of pituitary tumours induced by continuous oestrone stimulation and those induced by continuous thyroid hormone deprivation suggested a possible relationship between the two apparently different types of pituitary tumours in mice (chapter 3).

The observation that the thyroid weights in the oestrone treated mice were often twice the normal weight and in some cases even many times more (for example thyroid weights as high as 83 mg and 76 mg were found in castrated females $C_{57}Bl$; 71 mg in a castrated male ($C_{57}Bl \times DBA_f)F_1$) and 46 mg and 42 mg respectively in a male and a female ($O_{20} \times DBA_f)F_1$) suggested that information on the fluctuations of pituitary thyrotropin induced by the above mentioned procedures, during the period leading to tumour formation as well as information on the TSH content of the two types of pituitary tumours lead to a deeper understanding of this complex problem.

For this purpose it was necessary to develop a TSH-assay. Many species have been used for test animals. Most of the literature on this subject has been summarized by Wahlberg (1955) and Lameyer (1956). To avoid any difficulties due to possible species differences in pituitary hormones, mice were used exclusively as test animal for the thyrotropin assay. The assay method has been developed from a combination of the principles of the TSH-assay method used by van Eck (1940) and the method used by Querido, Kassenaar and Lameijer (1953) and has been described elsewhere (Kwa, 1959). It is based on the following principles: Endogenous TSH is allowed to reach near zero levels after surgical hypophysectomy; a series of equal doses of TSH at twelve hours intervals is then started to obtain a new "steady state" for the thyroid stimulation in the test animal. The 24 hrs uptake in the thyroid of a tracer dose of radioactive iodine administered together with the last hormone dose is considered as the index of stimulation caused by the administered hormone(s).

A. Substances in mouse pituitary homogenates interfering with a comparative TSH-assay

1. Data from the literature

Different reports have been published of the influence of other pituitary hormones on the action of thyrotropin on the thyroid. Noach (1953 and 1955) has proved that FSH (*f*ollicle *s*timulating *h*ormone) could enhance ^{131}I uptake in the thyroids of hypophysectomized female rats.

Presumably this was effected by inducing endogenous oestrone production in the ovaries of the test animals, for FSH had no effect on thyroidal ^{131}I uptake in spayed hypophysectomized rats.

It has been found that ACTH (*a*dreno *c*ortico*t*rophic *h*ormone) given concurrently inhibits the effect of a TSH dose in rats (MONEY, KRAINTZ, FAGER, KIRSCHNER and RAWSON, 1951; SOFFER, GABRILOVE and DORANCE, 1951; GABRILOVE, DORANCE and SOFFER, 1952; BROWN, WOODBURY, and SAYERS, 1952).

Adrenalectomy was reported to abolish the inhibitory effect of ACTH on TSH activity in rats (BROWN, et al., 1952), but ACTH has also been reported to decrease the TSH-induced ^{131}I accumulation in the thyroids of adrenalectomized animals (SOFFER, et al., 1951). The dosages used were rather massive and such quantities can not be expected to be contained in mouse pituitaries.

Our preliminary experiments were designed to find out whether crude mouse pituitary material contained any active principle(s) which could influence the end point of our TSH-assay sufficiently to complicate the interpretation of the results. Separation of different hormones by centrifugation of freshly prepared pituitary homogenate (HERLANT, 1952; BROWN and HESS, 1957) was preferred to chemical methods of isolating TSH. Current knowledge on the chemical properties of pituitary hormones is not sufficient to ensure that the percentage loss of TSH, which is risked when pituitary material is subjected to chemical isolation procedures will be the same in normal and pathological pituitaries.

From our preliminary experiments it appeared that mouse pituitaries contain at least two different active principles, which can influence TSH-induced uptake of ^{131}I in the thyroids of the test animals. Both principles can interfere with a comparative TSH-assay between the pituitaries of different strains of mice, as the pituitaries of different strains seem to contain these active principles in highly dissimilar quantities.

For the elucidation of this problem we made use of two observations.

a) The ^{131}I uptake by the thyroids of the test animals induced by a pituitary homogenate was different according as to whether total homogenate or the supernatant obtained by centrifuging the homogenate was injected. The effects were different on two genetically different *recipient* mice.

b) Castration of the recipient male testanimal had an effect on the ^{131}I uptake by the thyroid glands induced by pituitary homogenates. The effect of castration differed if the pituitaries used to make the pituitary homogenates were obtained from genetically different *donor* mice.

2. Materials and methods:

a) The recipient test animals were
$(O_{20} \times DBA_f)F_1$ designated as Od_f mice,
$(C_{57}Bl \times DBA_f)F_1$ designated as Bd_f mice and
C_3H mice, as indicated in the various experiments.

Male mice were hypophysectomized at the age of 6 to 10 weeks using the method of THOMAS (1938). In the experiments with gonadeectomized animals orchidectomy was done on the day of hypophysectomy or on the preceding day.

Body weights were controlled daily. Animals showing an increase in body weight compared with the pre-operative values were discarded. The animals were used for the assay eight to ten days after hypophysectomy. (In the following text "recipient mice" will always mean hypophysectomized mice, either castrated or non-castrated as designated).

b) Four equal doses of a pituitary homogenate, equivalent to $^1/_6$ of a mouse pituitary gland, were injected intra-peritoneally at twelve hour intervals.

c) Concurrently with the last dose, a tracer dose of radioactive iodine was given (0.10 ml of a stock solution, made for each experiment to approximately 10 μC/ml; carrier-free $Na^{131}I$ was purchased from Philips Roxane, Amsterdam).

d) The thyroid gland together with surrounding tissues, i.c. trachea and muscle covering, was dissected and homogenated in 30 to 40% NaOH. Radioactivity was measured in a liquid counter (20th Century, type: M 6 H). The radioactivity recovered was expressed as a percentage of the radioactivity of 0.10 ml of the stock solution used for the experiment. The value thus obtained was taken as the index of thyroid stimulation by the TSH contained in the injected dose of pituitary homogenate.

e) As pituitary donors the following mice have been used: male Od_f, male Bd_f and female and male of the F_1-hybrids ($WLL_f \times O_{20}$), designated as W_fO. Preparation of the pituitary homogenate: Donor mice were asphyxiated in ether, the skull cut open and the skull cap together with the cerebrum lifted up to expose the pituitary gland retained in its dural covering at the base of the skull. The dural covering was removed with fine watchmakers pincettes and the pituitary lifted in toto from the base of the skull with a small spoon and immediately transferred to ice-cold physiological saline (0.60 ml per pituitary).

f) The pooled pituitaries were homogenized in a mechanically driven Potter-Elvehjem homogenizer at 800 to 1,000 rpm, care being taken to ensure an adequate "fit" between the glasspounder and the glasstube. The resulting homogenate is called *total homogenate*. Centrifugation of pituitary homogenates:

1. Total homogenate was centrifuged in an uncooled outswinging Homef centrifuge at 2,500 × g for ten minutes. The slightly opalescent supernatant was used for injection.

2. Alternatively the supernatant was again centrifuged for sixty minutes at 18,000 × g at 0°—2° C in a Phywé-eispirouette, to yield a clear supernatant. The precipitates were discarded.

The time lapse between sacrificing the donor mice and the final separation of the supernatant should be as short as possible, (preferably less than one hour and a half in the case of centrifuging at 18,000 × g and less than half an hour in the other case).

3. Experiments

a) The choice of male mice as recipient animals. Pituitary gonadotrophins have been reported to influence ^{131}I uptake in female hypophysectomized rats (NOACH, 1953, 1955); presumably by inducing endogenous oestrone production. If this is also the case in mice, it would complicate the interpretation of a TSH-assay if female mice were used as recipient animals.

The results of a pilot experiment given in Table 9 suggest that in female mice the same mechanism as has been found in rats causes enhancement of ^{131}I uptake, the index for the stimulation of the thyroid by TSH in our assay.

We feel justified in using only male mice as recipient animals for our TSH-assay method because this ensures constancy of the endogenous oestrone level in the recipient animals in a comparative TSH-assay when the pituitary gonadotrophin content can be expected to vary in different pituitary donor groups.

Table 9. *^{131}I uptake induced in female recipient mice by the Sn 2,500 × g of pituitary homogenates. Influence of oestrone*

Donor	Mean percentage of ^{131}I uptake and standard error number of recipient mice per group in parentheses			p value (t test)
	Female Odf recipient	Spayed female Odf recipient	Spayed female Odf recipient, 0.1 γ oestrone concurrently	
female Odf in dioestrus	22.9 ± 0.7 (4)	13.2 ± 1.8 (4)		$p < 0.01$
male Odf	20.5 ± 1.4 (7)	20.0 ± 0.7[1] (4)	30.5 ± 3.1[1] (4)	$0.01 < p^1 < 0.02$

[1] The p value relates to the differences between these two groups.

b) The influence of centrifuging the homogenate at 2,500 × g. It was found that in Od_f recipient mice the administration of Sn 2,500 (the supernatant of a total homogenate centrifuged at 2,500 × g) resulted in a higher ^{131}I uptake by the thyroid compared with the uptake caused by the total homogenate (see Table 10).

The possibility that the lower TSH activity of total homogenate was caused by destruction of the hormone by proteolytic enzymes liberated when pituitary cells are crushed (SNYDER and SAYERS, 1953), became a less acceptable explanation of the observed difference between total homogenate and its Sn (2,500 × g), when it was found that the effect of centrifugation on ^{131}I uptake was reversed if Bd_f recipient mice were used (Table 11).

The possibility occurred to us that the interference with the ^{131}I uptake induced by TSH could be caused by an active principle in the total homogenate, which was precipitated by a centrifugal force of 2,500 × g. The opposite effects on TSH induced ^{131}I uptake by the

Table 10. *Influence of centrifuging pituitary homogenates (in Od_f recipents)*

Donor mice	Recipient mice	Mean percentage of ^{131}I uptake and standard error; no. of recipients in parentheses		p value (t test)
		Total homogenate	Sn (2,500 × g)	
male Od_f	male Od_f	10.3 ± 0.2 (3)	20.4 ± 1.9 (3)	$p < 0.01$
male Od_f	male Od_f castrated	16.1 ± 1.2 (3)	30.8 ± 2.6 (5)	$p < 0.01$
male Od_f	female Od_f	8.0 ± 0.5 (3)	20.5 ± 1.5 (7)	$p < 0.01$
female Od_f (dioestrus)	female Od_f	12.1 ± 0.2 (3)	22.9 ± 0.7 (4)	$p < 0.01$
female[1] Od_f	male Od_f castrated	13.2 ± 0.9 (5)	21.8 ± 1.4 (4)	$p < 0.01$
female[1] Od_f	male Od_f castrated 10 γ of cortisone	3.6 ± 0.3 (5)	9.6 ± 1.1 (5)	$p < 0.01$

[1] Randomly selected from cage, no vaginal smear taken, pituitaries pooled.

Table 11. *Influence of centrifuging pituitary homogenates (in Bd_f recipients)*

Donor mice	recipient mice	Mean percentage of ^{131}I uptake and standard error; no. of recipients in parentheses		p value (t test)
		Total homogenate	Sn (2,500 × g)	
male Bd_f	male Bd_f castrated	28.5 ± 1.2 (4)	10.0 ± 0.5 (4)	$p < 0.01$
male Bd_f	male Bd_f castrated 10 γ of cortisone	9.3 ± 0.7 (4)	6.7 ± 0.7 (4)	$0.02 < p < 0.05$
male Od_f	male Bd_f castrated	13.7 ± 1.9 (4)	8.3 ± 0.9 (4)	$0.02 < p < 0.05$
male Od_f	male Bd_f castrated 10 γ of cortisone	9.0 ± 1.5 (4)	6.1 ± 1.2 (4)	$0.10 < p < 0.20$

thyroids in recipient mice of these two particular strains, suggested the possibility of establishing the identity of such a principle.

According to HERLANT (1952) the granules presumed to contain ACTH are precipitated after centrifugation of a pituitary homogenate at the speed used.

Table 12, gives the results of the following experiment: a group of Od_f recipient mice and a group of Bd_f recipient mice were injected with lyophilized TSH obtained from Organon (batch no. 14,145, stated potency 0.79 USP/mg). The dose per injection was five micogram. The same dose was administered to two comparable groups of Od_f- and Bd_f-recipient mice concurrently with ACTH (8 μg of cortrophine, Organon commercial preparation). ACTH appeared to inhibit the TSH-induced ^{131}I uptake by the thyroids of the Od_f recipient mice, whereas it enhanced the ^{131}I uptake in the Bd_f recipient mice.

Table 12. *Different influence on TSH (ambinon, Organon) induced ^{131}I uptake in Bd_f- and Od_f-recipient mice of concurrent administration of ACTH (Cortrophine, Organon)*

Recipient mice	Mean percentage of ^{131}I uptake and standard error, number of recipient mice per group in parentheses		p value (t test)
	TSH + ACTH	TSH only	
castrated male Od_f, concurrently injected with 10 γ cortisone	7.5 ± 0.2 (5)	10.7 ± 0.4 (5)	$p < 0.01$
castrated male Bd_f, concurrently injected with 10 γ cortisone	9.3 ± 1.0 (5)	4.8 ± 0.3 (5)	$p < 0.01$

The parallelism between the effect of a lyophilized TSH preparation and the effect of the supernatant (2,500 × g) when compared to the effects of giving commercial ACTH concurrently with the lyophilized TSH preparation and of giving total homogenate respectively in these two differently reacting strains of mice used as recipient animals, suggests that the postulated active principle is either closely linked to ACTH or may be ACTH itself.

Further experiments using different strains of mice as pituitary donors suggested that the pituitaries of various strains contained this active principle in such dissimilar quantities that it prevented a reliable comparative TSH-assay by using total homogenate. It was decided therefore to use only the supernatant fraction of the homogenate for this purpose.

In both of the strains of mice used as recipient animals cortisone was found to have a depressive action on ^{131}I uptake by the thyroid. It was found, however, that a dose of 10 γ of cortisone injected concurrently with each administration of TSH permitted adequate precision in the assay of TSH (Kwa, 1959). The concurrent administration of this dose of cortisone was incorporated in the standardized TSH-assay method because it has the advantage of smoothing out any differences in the cortisone levels that might have been induced in the recipient animals by the ACTH remaining in the supernatant fraction of the pituitary homogenate used for the assay.

c) The effect of castration of the male recipient animals on thyroidal ^{131}I uptake. When it had been decided to use male mice as recipient animals for the TSH-assay, the possibility had to be investigated, whether in the male recipient mouse the TSH-induced ^{131}I uptake by the thyroid was influenced by the pituitary gonadotrophins through an induction of gonadal hormone production, as was suggested to be the case in female mice by the results of our pilot experiment. Experiments with male mice indicated that castration enhanced ^{131}I uptake by the thyroid induced by pituitary homogenate administration (Table 13).

A higher ^{131}I uptake by the thyroid gland in castrated recipient mice compared to non-castrated ones was observed in Od_f mice, either injected with total homogenate, or with the supernatant (2,500 × g) fraction. The observed difference in ^{131}I uptake between castrated and non-castrated recipient mice persisted when cortisone was given concurrently

Table 13. *Influence of castration of the recipient mice on their thyroidal* ^{131} *I uptake*

Donor mice	Recipient mice	Mean percentage ^{131}I uptake and standard error; no. of recipients in parentheses		p value (t test)
		castrated	non-castrated	
male Odf (total homogenate)	male Odf	16.1 ± 1.2 (3)	10.3 ± 0.2 (3)	$p < 0.01$
male Odf (Sn 2,500)	male Odf	28.7 ± 2.8 (4)	13.0 ± 1.2 (5)	$p < 0.01$
male Odf (Sn 2,500)	male Odf 10 γ of cortisone	8.6 ± 0.5 (5)	6.3 ± 0.8 (3)	$0.02 < p < 0.05$
male Odf (F_2) (Sn 2,500)	male Odf 10 γ of cortisone	6.8 ± 0.3 (4)	5.2 ± 0.6 (4)	$p \pm 0.05$
male Odf (Sn 2,500)	male Bdf 10 γ of cortisone	12.8 ± 1.2 (6)	9.6 ± 0.4 (4)	$p \pm 0.05$
male Odf (F_2) (Sn 2,500)	male Bdf 10 γ of cortisone	6.2 ± 0.2 (4)	3.6 ± 0.3 (3)	$p < 0.01$

with the supernatant fraction. In Bd_f mice, in which cortisone was given concurrently in all experiments, the difference between castrated and non-castrated recipients was also observed (Table 13).

Further pilot-experiments in which either testosterone, oestrone or progestrone was injected concurrently with the pituitary homogenate did not reveal an inhibitory action of these hormones on ^{131}I uptake by the thyroid. The mechanism of the enhancement of the ^{131}I uptake by the thyroid caused by castration of the recipient animal remained obscure. The increased sensitivity obtained with the castrated recipient mice and the exclusion of a possible effect of gonadotrophins on the end point of our assay through the induction of gonadal hormone production suggested the use of castrated male mice as recipients.

d) A second interfering substance. It was found that pituitary homogenates from certain donor strains induced a *lower* ^{131}I uptake by the thyroid in *castrated recipients* than in non-castrated ones.

The consequence of this observation for a comparative assay of pituitary homogenates of the apparently different types is illustrated by the ^{131}I uptake results represented in Table 14.

The ^{131}I uptake effected by the administration of two different pituitary homogenates into groups of recipient mice of the same genetic constitution can be considered to reflect the TSH content of the two pituitaries under examination, provided that the homogenates do not contain other hormones or active principles influencing the end point of the assay in such different amounts as to interfere with the comparative TSH-assay. Repeating the comparative assay using either another strain or using castrated instead of non-castrated mice as the recipient animals should then yield the same estimate of the relative TSH potencies of the two pituitaries tested.

However, the ^{131}I uptakes by the thyroid induced in the recipient mice by Od_f- and W_fO-pituitaries do not permit an unequivocal conclusion as to which type of pituitary contained the more TSH. The ^{131}I uptakes induced by Od_f-homogenates and by W_fO-homogenates differed according to the type of recipient animal. In some mice both homogenates produced the same results; in others the Od_f-homogenate produced a greater effect than W_fO-homogenate and in others again it produced a smaller effect (see Table 14).

Table 14. *The difference in thyroidal* ^{131}I *uptake in castrated and non-castrated recipient mice appeared to be dependent on pituitary donor strain.* (N. B. Thyroidal ^{131}I uptake in C_3H recipient mice appeared not to be influenced by castration)

Recipent mice	Mean percentage of ^{131}I uptake and standard error; no. of recipients in parentheses, p value difference: castrates non-castrates		Inference on TSH content of the two pituitariies
	W_fO (Sn 2,500)	Od_f (F_2) (Sn 2,500)	
Bdf non-castrated	6.1 ± 0.8 (3)	3.6 ± 0.3 (3)	$W_fO > Od_f$ (F_2)
Bdf castrated	2.7 ± 0.8 (5)	6.2 ± 0.3 (4)	$W_fO < Od_f$ (F_2)
	$0.02 < p < 0.05$	$0.02 < p < 0.05$	
Odf non-castrated	7.8 ± 0.3 (3)	5.2 ± 0.6 (4)	$W_fO > Od_f$ (F_2)
Odf castrated	5.8 ± 0.3 (4)	6.8 ± 0.3 (4)	$W_fO \leqq Od_f$ (F_2)
	$0.01 < p < 0.02$	$0.02 < p < 0.05$	
C_3H non-castrated	12.7 ± 0.3 (3)	6.6 ± 0.6 (6)	$W_fO > Od_f$ (F_2)
C_3H castrated	11.9 ± 0.7 (3)	6.1 ± 0.6 (4)	$W_fO > Od_f$ (F_2)
	$0.20 < p < 0.30$	$0.50 < p < 0.60$	

In Od_f-as well as in Bd_f-recipient mice the castrated recipients showed a higher ^{131}I uptake than the non-castrated ones when injected with Od_f pituitary homogenate. This response was called the Od_f-effect. The W_fO pituitary homogenate elicited the reverse response, the castrated recipients showing a lower ^{131}I uptake than the non-castrated ones. This was called the W_fO-effect. If there is an unidentified active principle in one of the pituitary homogenates responsible for the different effect it should be possible by injecting the principle concurrently with the pituitary homogenate to obtain either a W_fO-effect with an Od_f pituitary homogenate, or an Od_f-effect with a W_fO pituitary homogenate, depending on which of the two homogenates already has the active principle in excess. The weights of the testes and the seminal vesicles induced by the two types of pituitary homogenates in the non-castrated recipient Bd_f mice (Table 15) indicated a considerable difference in the gonadotrophic hormone content, the W_fO pituitaries containing more FSH and LH.

Table 15

Sn (2,500 × g)	Bd-recipients no. of mice	Organ weights in mg	
		Testes ± st. err.	Prostate ± st. err.
W_fO pituitary	4	165.2 ± 8.8	6.2 ± 0.2
Od_f pituitary	4	91.5 ± 15.8	2.8 ± 0.5
physiol. saline	4	45.4 ± 5.5	1.7 ± 0.6

In a series of pilot experiments a variety of other known pituitary hormones were injected concurrently with either of the two pituitary homogenates. The results indicated, that it was possible to obtain a W_fO-effect when an Od_f pituitary homogenate was injected concurrently with prolactin (Organon, batch Res. P. 175) in Od_f- as well as in Bd_f-recipient mice.

The results of a typical experiment are represented in Table 16: Od_f homogenate was centrifuged at 2,500 × g; the supernatant was injected into four groups of castrated and four groups of non-castrated Bd_f recipient mice. The first pair of the groups was injected in addition with physiological saline, the other pairs with 0.5, 1.0 and 2.0 IU. respectively of prolactin concurrently with each pituitary homogenate administration.

Table 16. *Influence of prolactin (Organon) on ^{131}I uptake in Bd_f recipient mice induced by $Od_f(F_2)$ pituitary homogenate*

Sn (2,500) pituitary donor	Dose of prolactin in IU	^{131}I uptake, mean percentage and standard error, no. of recipient mice in parentheses; all recipient mice injected with 10 γ cortisone		Statistical significance student's t-test
		castrated	non-castrated	p value
Od_f (F_2)	0.0 (phys. sal.)	6.3 ± 0.2 (5)	4.8 ± 0.5 (4)	$0.01 < p < 0.02$
Od_f (F_2)	0.5	6.1 ± 0.3 (4)	6.0 ± 0.5 (5)	$0.90 < p$
Od_f (F_2)	1.0	4.9[1] ± 0.2 (4)	6.4 ± 0.6 (4)	$0.02 < p < 0.05$
Od_f (F_2)	2.0	3.5[1] ± 0.2 (4)	6.4 ± 0.7 (5)	$p < 0.01$

[1] Decrease of ^{131}I uptake due to prolactin dose statistically significant at $p < 0.01$ level.

The reduction in the percentage uptake of ^{131}I in the castrated recipient mice effected by the two highest doses of prolactin compared with the physiological saline group is statistically significant. The increase in the ^{131}I uptake in the non-castrated groups receiving the prolactin doses compared with the group receiving physiological saline concurrently with the pituitary homogenate, appeared not to be statistically significant. A typical Od_f-effect was shown by the pair of groups (castrated compared with "intact") receiving the Od_f-homogenate and in addition the physiological saline, while the two pairs of groups of the series receiving the two highest dosages of prolactin showed the typical W_fO-effect. (The difference between the ^{131}I uptake of the castrated and the non-castrated recipient mice in all pairs of groups mentioned was statistically significant).

It had been reported that prolactin (luteotropin) activity (HERLANT, 1952) was found only in the sediment fraction, the supernatant fraction showing practically no activity in the biological test used. The possibility that the gravitational force resulting from centrifugation at 2,500 × g as used thus far in our experiments, had not been sufficient to spin out prolactin activity was investigated next.

Results of a typical experiment in which a far greater centrifugal speed was used (18,000 × g being the maximum centrifugal force available), are represented in Table 17.

Table 17. *Difference in ^{131}I uptake induced by the same W_fO pituitary homogenate in castrated Bd_f recipient mice between the aliquot Sn (2,500 × g) used for the injections as such and the aliquot again centrifuged and its Sn (18,000 × g) used for the injections*

Bd_f recipient mice concurrently injected 10γ of cortisone	Mean percentage ^{131}I uptake and standard error, number of recipients in parentheses		Student's t-test
	Sn (2,500 × g)	Sn (18,000 × g)	p value
castrated	2.2 ± 0.7 (6)	12.4 ± 1.0 (5)	$p < 0.01$
non-castrated	8.4 ± 1.0 (6)	8.8 ± 0.7 (6)	$0.60 < p < 0.70$
p value:	$p < 0.01$	$p < 0.01$	

Freshly prepared ♀ W_fO-homogenate was centrifuged at 2,500 × g (♀ W_fO were used as pituitary donor mice in this experiment as it was found during the preliminary experiments that the pituitaries of female mice of this strain gave a more clearcut "W_fO-effect" than pituitaries of males). Aliquots of the supernatant were used for a series of injections into two groups of Bd_f recipient mice (castrated and "intact" groups), the remainder of the supernatant (2,500 × g) was again centrifuged at 18,000 × g. The 18,000 × g supernatant was used for the series of injections into the two corresponding groups of recipient mice.

The results showed that the 2,500 × g supernatant of the W_fO-pituitary homogenate gave the typical "W_fO-effect", but the 18,000 × g supernatant obtained by centrifuging an aliquot of the 2,500 × g supernatant gave the typical "Od_f-effect". Apparently this "conversion" had been effected by an increase of the ^{131}I uptake in the castrated recipient mice. It must be inferred that the centrifugal force separated an active principle from the 18,000 × g supernatant containing the TSH and that this principle develops its greatest depressive action on ^{131}I uptake in the castrated animal This observation excluded the possibility that the depressive action on thyroid uptake of ^{131}I is mediated through the induction of gonadal hormone production. It made a concept of the mechanism by which it interferes rather difficult to viusalize.

However, for the practical aspects of the problem of assaying thyrotropin the preliminary experiments have yielded useful information.

4. Conclusions:

a) The mouse pituitary appears to contain at least two different active principles influencing thyroid uptake of ^{131}I induced in the recipient test animals by TSH.

The first appears to be either closely linked to ACTH or to be ACTH itself; it influences ^{131}I uptake in the castrated and in the "intact" recipient mice about equally. The second appears to be closely linked to prolactin or may be prolactin itself. It decreases thyroid uptake of ^{131}I in the castrated recipient mice to a far greater extent than in non-castrated test animals.

b) For a comparative TSH assay to give reliable information on the ratios of the actual TSH contents of pituitaries from different donor groups it is imperative to separate the TSH from the two active principles in the assay material. For this purpose centrifugation of the freshly prepared pituitary homogenate may be used. This method of separation has the advantage that it is relatively "gentle" in comparison to chemical methods of separation, this being especially important in view of the protein nature of the pituitary hormones. It ensures that the thyroid stimulating activity of the native TSH is being assayed and not that of any possible, chemically produced artefacts with thyroid-stimulating properties. A comparative TSH-assay using centrifuged pituitary homogenate can therefore be relied upon not to produce false high values for thyrotropin. Centrifugation shares with all other purification methods the risk of losing an unknown percentage of TSH. A drawback specific to the method is that one can never be certain of having separated all of each of the interfering substances. In fact the separation by centrifugation can not be expected to be 100% effective as centrifugation will only separate the fraction of any water soluble protein, that is contained in sub-cellular structures. The fraction that is either not contained in sub-cellular structures, or has diffused out of the precipitable granules during the process (i. e the fraction that has dissolved into the physiological saline) cannot be separated by centrifugation with the centrifugal force used. For these reasons false low values for TSH, caused either by partial loss of the hormone or by a failure to separate the inhibiting substances from the homogenate used for the assay cannot be excluded.

B. Comparative assays of the TSH content of pituitaries of mice treated in various ways to induce pituitary tumours development

1. Data from the literature

a) The possible action of oestrone on thyroid physiology and TSH content of the pituitary. The modifying actions of oestrogens on the thyroid have been generally recognized. The effect on basal metabolism was first described by LAQUEUR, HART and DE JONGH (1926) and confirmed by many others (TAGLIAFERRO, 1933; PINCUS and WERTHESSEN, 1933; SHERWOOD, 1936). Small doses of oestrogen given during short periods raise the basal metabolism, whereas more massive doses, or oestrogen given over prolonged periods lower the basal metabolism. Changes in thyroid weights are reported to correspond with changes in the metabolic rate. More massive doses and prolonged treatment, however, do not always result in a decrease of thyroid weight: The relatively high dose of 50 I U. of oestradiol daily for 24 days (DESCLIN and ERMANS, 1950) increased thyroid weights in rats and the long-term experiments in the Netherlands Cancer Institute oestrone increased these weights in most strains of mice as well as in rats.

The reports on the modifying action of oestrogen on the physiology of the thyroid gland as reflected in different functional criteria also appear to be equivocal, since oestrogens have been reported: not to influence ^{131}I uptake in spayed female rats (PASCHKIS, CANTAROW and PEACOCK, 1948); to slow down the turnover rate of ^{131}I in chicks (EPSTEIN and WOLTERINK, 1949) and to inhibit the effect of TSH on the thyroid of the guinea pig (NOVELLI, 1952).

The level at which oestrogens exert their modifying action seems also to be in dispute: It has been supposed to stimulate the anterior lobe of the pituitary and enhance TSH secretion (FREUDENBERGER and CLAUSEN, 1937; CALAPA, 1950; DESCLIN and ERMANS, 1950); a modifying action of oestradiol acting at the thyroid level has been proved by NOACH (1953, 1955), whereas the experiments of CLIFTON and MEYER (1956 a) appear to disclose its action at the pituitary gland level; DESCLIN (1952) inferred that the thyroid hypertrophy was the result of a neutralizing effect of oestrogens on thyroxin-like products of the thyroid.

From the literature it appears that oestrogen modifies thyroid physiology and morphology, probably acting at the thyroid gland level as well as at the pituitary level. The possibility that the presumed enhancement of TSH secretion is caused by an interference with the normal servo control between thyroid and pituitary has been inferred.

When the preliminary experiments in developing a TSH-assay method for the present investigation suggested that prolactin excess could inhibit the thyroid uptake of ^{131}I induced by TSH (see V. A. 2. d.), it was appreciated that prolonged oestrone administration to the intact mouse may interfere with thyroid hormone synthesis by inducing an excessive secretion of prolactin. This excess of prolactin, by inhibiting the normal TSH-controlled iodine uptake in the thyroid gland, may be conceived to lower thyroid hormone production and thus indirectly cause the TSH producing cells of the pituitary to react according to the servo mechanism to the thyroid hormone deficiency.

b) The effect of thyroid hormone deprivation on pituitary TSH. According to current opinion the pituitary reacts to deprivation of thyroid hormone induced by thyroidectomy, etc., with an increased TSH secretion, an increase in the size, and probably (although only in the mouse) with an increase in the number of the cells producing the hormone (GRIESBACH and PURVES, 1943; PURVES and GRIESBACH 1951 a and b, 1957; HALMI, 1952 a and b; HALMI and GUDE, 1954).

SEVERINGHAUS (1937) stressed the theoretical possibility that cytological and histological evidence of hyperfunction of a hormone-producing pituitary cell could well be reconciled with physiological evidence of a decreased pituitary content of the hormone involved (assay results, etc.) It could even be reconciled with additional physiological evidence of normal or sub-normal blood levels of that hormone (parabiosis experiments, assay results, etc.), since the increase in the rate of release of the hormone from the pituitary gland may exceed the increased production so that a depletion of the quantity of stored hormone results. When in addition a rapid destruction, inactivation or excretion of the hormone takes place, no detectable rise in the blood level will appear.

On the basis of investigations into the effects of thyroid hormone deficiency and thyroid hormone excess on the TSH content of the pituitary GRIESBACH and PURVES, (1943, 1945; PURVES and GRIESBACH, 1951 a and b) designated the angular, periodic acid Schiff positive (PAS) and aldehyde-fuchsin positive basophile pituitary cell as the TSH-producing cell. HALMI first designated the aldehyde-fuchsin negative, PAS-positive "delta" basophile cell as the probable site of TSH production (1950), but later revised his conclusion and agreed with PURVES and GRIESBACH that the "beta" basophile cell is the TSH producing cell. HALMI made the following interesting remark (1952 b): "... this reasoning obviously hinges on the assumption that the findings of GRIESBACH and PURVES concerning thyrotropin content of the pituitary in hypothyroidism and athyroidism are correct ...". and drew attention to the fact that the data from the literature on this subject do not appear to be unequivocal. Whereas the decrease in pituitary TSH content after thyroxin treatment appears to be well founded (HOHLWEG and JUNKMAN, 1933; KUSCHINSKY, 1933; GRIESBACH and PURVES, 1945; MC QUILLAN, TRIKOJUS, CAMPBELL and TURNER, 1948), pituitary TSH contents after thyroidectomy have been reported to be: substantially decreased per unit weight (GRIESBACH and PURVES, 1943); slightly decreased per unit weight, but increased per whole gland (ZECKWER, 1936); slightly decreased per whole gland (LEBEDEWA, 1936; TURNER and CUPPS, 1940); practically unchanged (HOUSSAY, NOVELLI and SAMMARTINO, 1932; HOHLWEG and JUNKMAN, 1933); and slightly increased (CH'EN and VAN DYKE, 1936; TURNER and CUPP, 1940; MERCIER-PAROT and TUCHMANN-DUPLESSIS, 1954). TURNER and CUPPS (1940) reported a sex difference: male thyroidectomized rats showed a slight decrease, female thyroidectomized rats a slight increase in pituitary TSH content. All the observers used rats as pituitary donor animals with the exception of CH'EN and VAN DYKE, who used rabbits. HOUSSAY et al. used guinea-pigs, dogs and toads as experimental pituitary donor animals as well as rats.

In mice the pituitary TSH content appears to increase after thyroid destruction (FURTH, DENT, BURNETT and GADSDEN, 1955). The pituitary tumours induced in mice in this way have been reported to have approximately the same TSH content per unit weight as normal mouse pituitaries (BATES, ANDERSON and FURTH, 1957).

The opinions about the effect of thyroidectomy on the blood level of TSH appear to be equally equivocal. Evidence of an enhanced TSH secretion could not be demonstrated by parabiosis experiments, when a thyroidectomized rat was united with an intact partner (HOUSSAY, 1932; PUMMEAU-DELILLE, 1948). Evidence of an increased TSH secretion was obtained, however, when a thyroidectomized rat was united to a hypophysectomized partner with an intact thyroid gland (KONEFF, VAN DYKE and EVANS, 1952). The description of normal acidophile cells in the pituitary of the thyroidectomized animal by KONEFF et al. may be interpreted as an indication that thyroid hormone of the hypophysectomized partner has entered the circulation of the thyroidectomized rat in sufficient amounts to cause regranulation of the acidophile cells. The finding of acidophile cells in the pituitary of thyroidectomized rats has been described as an infallible sign of incomplete removal of the thyroid gland (LEBEDEWA, 1936; GRIESBACH and PURVES, 1943). It may be inferred that parabiosis experiments are not suitable for the study of the effect of thyroidectomy on the blood level of TSH. Attempts to assay TSH in the blood of thyroidectomized rats have been numerous. GRIESBACH and PURVES reported a substantial and statistically significant increase, but could not give an estimate of the percentage increase, since the response elicited with the blood of normal rats was not on the straight portion of the dose-response curve of their assay method (1943). DEL CONTE and STUX (1955), using their very sensitive assay based on intra-cellular colloid droplets in the guinea-pig's thyroid, reported a 500fold increase in the blood level of TSH of thyroidectomized rats as compared with untreated control rats. It is of interest that they ascribe the failure of others (D'ANGELO, GORDON and CHARIPPER, 1942; GORDON, GOLDSMITH and CHARIPPER, 1945; D'ANGELO, 1953 and 1954), who used the very sensitive tadpole technique, to their use of total serum, thus omitting a separation of TSH from supposed interfering substances. The intracellular colloid droplet assay method, however, is stated to be almost certainly not specific for TSH (LORAINE, 1958).

The blood levels of TSH of mice bearing grafts of pituitary tumours, which had been induced by a thyroid-destructive dose of radioactive iodine, have been reported to show a considerable increase, which is stated to parallel the tumour mass of "thyrotropes" (BATES, ANDERSON and FURTH, 1957).

A survey of the literature showed that the reported data about the effect of thyroidectomy on the pituitary content, as well as on the blood level, of TSH in the rat are contradictory. In the mouse thyroidectomy appears to increase the pituitary content as well as the blood level of TSH.

2. Material and methods

Pituitary assay material:

Eighty male (C_{57}Bl × C_3H_f) F_1 mice, designated as BC_3H_f, were castrated at the age of two to three months and distributed randomly into four groups: one group of twenty mice received no treatment and served as control pituitary donors, the other three groups received the various treatments used to induce pituitary tumours at the Netherland's Cancer Institute. The first group of twenty mice was given a thyroid-destructive dose of radioactive iodine, the second group was put on the methylthiouracil regimen, and the third group was put on the oestrone-regimen (see III., 1. b.).

After an interval of 6 weeks, four comparable groups of another hybrid, (C_{57}Bl × DBA_f) F_1 were started. Pituitary hormones are of protein nature and theoretically "foreign-protein reactions" may interfere with a bio-assay of any of these hormones. The decision to include this hybrid as a pituitary donor was based on the consideration that it would provide a "theoretically ideal bio-assay", since the recipient test animals used in the assays were of the same genetic constitution.

After another six weeks interval four additional groups of BC_3H_f mice, consisting of five mice each, were started in a repeat experiment.

At stated time intervals after starting treatment five mice were randomly chosen from each treatment group for a comparative assay of the TSH content of their pituitaries. The mice were injected with a tracer dose of radioactive iodine and were killed the following day. The thyroids of the donor animals were dissected as has been described for the recipient animals (see V. A. 2. d.) to obtain information on the functional state of the glands. The five pituitaries of the mice from each treatment group were pooled in ice-cold physiological saline and prepared for the TSH-assay as described (see V. A. 2. f.), except that the largest centrifugal force used was not 18,000 $\times$ g as described for the preliminary assays, but was accidentally 24,000 $\times$ g in the first three assay series and in the subsequent assay series it was set at 14,000 $\times$ g.

As recipient test animals ($C_{57}Bl \times DBA_f$) F_1 hybrid mice were used exclusively in all assays. The test animals were injected with 10 γ of cortisone concurrently with each administration of the pituitary homogenate (see V. A. 3. b.). In the first three series only castrated recipient mice were used. In the next four series the pituitary homogenates were tested simultaneously on eight groups of castrated and eight groups of "intact" mice. In the last two series eight groups of "intact" and four groups of castrated mice were used.

The comparative assay was planned as a "four times two-point" assay; namely for each assay series used to compare four types of pituitary homogenates, forty recipient mice were divided into eight groups of five mice each. For each pituitary homogenate two groups were used: The five mice of one group received the equivalent of 1/12 (or 1/6 as stated) of a pituitary per injection, the five mice of the other group received the equivalent of 1/60 of a pituitary per injection. In the assay of the pituitaries of Bd_f mice eleven months after initiation of treatment, the high dose (1/12 of a pituitary per injection) was omitted and two additional groups received the equivalents of 1/300 and 1/1500 of a pituitary per injection respectively.

The ratios between the TSH content of each of the homogenates of pooled pituitaries of the treated donor groups and the TSH content of the homogenate of pooled pituitaries of the control group was calculated by the method of GADDUM (1953)[1] from the ^{131}I uptake induced in the thyroids of the recipient mice.

[1] Since only the high dose of the "control homogenate" in each of the series of assays induced a thyroid ^{131}I uptake that could be considered to fall on the straight part of the dose-response curve, the ratios were calculated on the basis of a "three point" assay. This could only be done for those homogenates, which in both concentrations employed induced ^{131}I uptakes by the thyroid that could be considered to fall on the straight part of the dose-response curve. All sets of such "two-points" within a series performed on the same day were considered to add information on the variance of the slope of the particular assay series. When only one, two or three sets of "two-points" were considered to fall on the straight part of the dose-response curve, the variance of the slope was considered to be $2V/I^2$, V/I^2 or $2V/3I^2$ respectively.

3. Results:

a) Assay series using the Sn 24,000 × g of the pituitary homogenates. The results of the first three comparative assay series, in which the homogenates used for the assays had been centrifuged at the maximum speed of the Phywe are given in Table 18.

Table 18

Strain of donor mouse duration of treatment	Pituitary dose level used, comparative TSH value, etc.	Assay results using castrated hypophysectomized mice as recipient animals to compare the TSH content of four groups donor pituitaries, five pituitaries of each donor group were pooled and homogenized in physiological saline and the Sn 24,000 g used as assay material				
		control %	oestrone %	$Na^{131}I$ %	MTU %	λ
BC_3HfF_1 $2^1/_2$ week	1/ 6 pit. aeq./inj.	4.4	4.1	1.6	20.5	0.149
	1/60 pit. aeq./inj.	—	1.1	1.2	8.8	
	comp. TSH value	*100*	± *100*	< *40*	*2260*	
	5% fiduc. upper:	—	—	—	3864	
	limits lower:	—	—	—	1677	
	individual slopes[1]	—	—	—	(11.7)	
BC_3HfF_1 7 weeks	1/6 pit. aeq./inj..	10.1	8.2	19.2	4.4	0.143
	1/60 pit. aeq./inj.	—	0.9	5.2	1.0	
	comp. TSH value	*100*	± *75*	*446*	± *40*	
	5% fiduc. upper:	—	—	775	—	
	limits lower:	—	—	269	—	
	individual slopes[1]	—	—	(14.0)	—	
$BdfF_1$ $2^1/_2$ week	1/ 6 pit. aeq./inj.	2.9	2.1	0.9	3.4	—
	1/60 pit. aeq./inj.	—	1.1	0.9	1.1	
	comp. TSH value	*100*	≦ *100*	< *20*	≧ *100*	
	5% fiduc. upper:	—	—	—	—	
	limits lower:	—	—	—	—	
	individual slopes[1]	—	—	—	—	

[1] The values for individual slopes are not expressed in percent.

From the first comparative TSH assay series, BC_3H_f mice killed $2^1/_2$ week after beginning treatment, only the homogenate of the pituitaries from the methylthiouracil treated animals resulted in thyroid uptakes of ^{131}I in both concentrations used (1/6 and 1/60 of a pituitary per injection respectively) that could be considered to fall well within the straight portion of the dose-response curve. The TSH content of the pituitary in the methylthiouracil treated donor mice was calculated to have increased to 22.6 times the content of that in the untreated mice (5% fiducial limits 16.8—38.6). The thyroid uptake of ^{131}I induced in the recipient mice by "oestrone pituitary" homogenate was nearly the same as that induced by the "control pituitary" homogenate. The "radiothyroidectomy pituitary" homogenate resulted in an uptake in the recipient mice, which did not differ from the thyroid uptake in the recipient mice injected with physiological saline.

In the second series comprising BC_3H_f mice 7 weeks after initiation of treatment, the "methylthiouracil pituitary" homogenate resulted in a statistically significant lower thyroid uptake of ^{131}I in the recipient mice compared with the "control pituitary" homogenate. The TSH content may be estimated to be approximately 40% of the control value or less. The "oestrone pituitary" homogenate appeared to be slightly lower in TSH potency than the "control pituitary" homogenate but the induced ^{131}I uptake in the recipient mice did not differ significantly. The "radiothyroidectomy pituitary" homogenate was calculated to have been 4.5 times the TSH potency of the "control pituitary" homogenate (5% fiducial limits: 2.7—7.75).

The thyroid uptakes of ^{131}I were very low for all four of the pooled pituitary homogenates in the third comparative assay series comprising Bd_f donor mice killed $2^1/_2$ week after initiation of treatment. The uptake induced by the "methylthiouracil pituitary" homogenate was slightly higher, and the uptake induced by the "oestrone pituitary" homogenate lower than that induced by the "control pituitary" homogenate but the differences were not statistically significant. The difference between the uptake induced by the "methylthiouracil pituitary" homogenate and by the "oestrone pituitary" homogenate was significant at the $0.02 < p < 0.05$ level. The thyroid ^{131}I uptakes induced in the recipient mice by the "radiothyroidectomy pituitary" homogenate again did not differ from the thyroid uptake of ^{131}I in the recipient mice injected with physiological saline.

The ^{131}I uptake induced by the homogenate of pituitaries of untreated Bd_f donor mice was lower than was expected from previous experience. In the preliminary experiments thyroid uptake of ^{131}I induced by homogenates of Bd_f pituitaries in recipient mice of the same strain had always been about twice as high as was found in the present experiment. The various steps in the assay procedure were examined and it was found that the maximal centrifugal force of the centrifuge had increased from the previous $18{,}000 \times g$ to $24{,}000 \times g$. This increase could be attributed to replacement of the electrical power main two months previously. The unintended use of a larger centrifugal force probably had disturbed the comparative TSH-assays and the possibility was considered whether the extremely low TSH content of the Sn $24{,}000 \times g$ homogenates of the "radiothyroidectomy pituitaries" found in BC_3H_f- and Bd_f-strains at $2^1/_2$ weeks after starting treatment were caused by a loss of TSH in the discarded precipitate. The considerable difference in TSH content found between the Sn $24{,}000 \times g$ of the BC_3H_f "methylthiouracil pituitary" homogenates at $2^1/_2$ week and at 7 weeks after starting treatment also may have been caused artificially and only reflect a difference in percentage loss between the two assays.

In view of the theoretical possibility of "coarser" TSH-containing granules in the experimental pituitaries it was decided to use a somewhat lower centrifugal force than in the preliminary experiments and lessen the chance of losing TSH from the supernatants. For the subsequent assays a centrifugal force of $14{,}000 \times g$ was used. The comparative assay of BC_3H_f pituitaries at $2^1/_2$ week after starting treatment was repeated with the lower centrifugal force.

Tab-

Strain of donor mouse duration of treatment	24-hrs. uptake of ^{131}I in thyroids of donor mice at time of sacrifice, (mean of four animals per group)				Assay results using hypo- of each donor groups were
	control %	oestrone %	$Na^{131}I$ %	MTU %	Pituitary dose level used, comparative TSH value, etc.
BC_3HfF_1 2½ week	15.9	13.1	2.6	16.0	1/12 pit. aeq./inj. 1/60 pit. aeq./inj. comp. TSH value 5% fiduc. upper: limits lower: individual slopes
BC_3HfF_1 25 weeks	16.9	16.8	0.8	12.3	1/12 pit. aeq./inj. 1/60 pit. aeq./inj. comp. TSH value 5% fiduc. upper: limits lower: individualslopes
BC_3HfF_1 53 weeks	17.5	23.3	0.6	12.9	1/12 pit. aeq./inj. 1/60 pit. aeq./inj. comp. TSH value 5% fiduc. upper: limits lower: individual slopes
$BdfF_1$ 9 weeks	41.8	28.9	0.7	39.8	1/12 pit. aeq./inj. 1/60 pit. aeq./inj. comp. TSH value 5% fiduc. upper: limits lower: individual slopes
$BdfF_1$ 23 weeks	46.6	15.2	0.7	39.3	1/12 pit. aeq./inj. 1/60 pit. aeq./inj. comp. TSH value 5% fiduc. upper: limits lower: individual slopes
$BdfF_1$ 46 weeks	26.4	53.3	0.7	12.1	1/12 pit. aeq./inj. 1/60 pit. aeq./inj. 1/300 pit. aeq./inj. 1/1500 pit. aeq./inj. comp. TSH value 5% fiduc. upper: limits lower: individual slopes

[1] The dosages of the assay material injected had been too potent, the induced reflected in the flattening of the individual slope and the great dispersion shown by

b) Assay series using the Sn 14,000 × g of pituitary homogenates. The use of a smaller centrifugal force than had been proved to separate the second interfering principle sufficiently from the TSH-containing supernatant for assay purposes, involved the risk of a less complete separation

le 19

physectomized mice to compare the TSH content of the four groups of donor pituitaries, four pituitaries pooled and homogenized in physiological saline, the Sn 14,000 g were assayed simultaneously in castrated recipient mice as well as in non-castrated recipient mice.

24 hrs. ^{131}I uptake induced, calculated comparative TSH values (control = 100%), etc.									
results in non-castrated recipient mice:					results in castrated recipient mice:				
control %	oestrone %	$Na^{131}I$ %	MTU %	λ	control %	oestrone %	$Na^{131}I$ %	MTU %	λ
2.5	1.0	8.7	9.6	0.077	3.1	1.1	9.6	10.5	0.052
—	0.8	2.4	2.0		—	0.9	1.6	2.4	
100	*≦40*	*452*	*480*		*100*	*≦40*	*368*	*436*	
—	—	614	653		—	—	443	523	
—	—	345	367		—	—	307	367	
—	—	(9.0)	(10.9)		—	—	(11.4)	(11.6)	
1.6	2.0	9.7	12.5	0.068	1.9	1.7	10.6	11.4	0.084
—	0.7	2.4	4.6		—	0.8	4.4	5.0	
100	*±100*	*565*	*953*		*100*	*±100*	*933*	*1116*	
—	—	748	1337		—	—	1498	1789	
—	—	429	710		—	—	680	822	
—	—	(10.4)	(11.3)		—	—	(8.9)	(9.2)	
7.0	6.9	47.2[1]	23.9	0.161	4.1	6.4	34.9	31.9	—
—	—	42.4[1]	16.9		—	—	—	—	
100	*±100*	*'1795200'*	*5100*		*100*	*≧100*	*≫100*	*≫100*	
—	—	'35693570'	34001		—	—	—	—	
—	—	'47390'	1701		—	—	—	—	
—	—	(6.9[1])	(10.0)		—	—	—	—	
3.0	10.9	19.1	20.8	0.169	6.1	6.3	19.7	20.8	0.123
—	3.6	10.3	11.1		—	—	13.6	11.5	
100	*503*	*2158*	*2665*		*100*	*±100*	*1978*	*1860*	
—	935	4498	5651		—	—	3023	2833	
—	277	1342	1669		—	—	1490	1398	
—	(10.4)	(12.6)	(13.9)		—	—	(8.7)	(13.3)	
3.1	9.5	15.9	20.4	0.134	6.4	6.0	18.4	16.7	0.105
—	3.5	7.6	13.1		—	—	9.1	7.5	
100	*477*	*1542*	*4714*		*100*	*±100*	*804*	*603*	
—	841	3139	12009		—	—	1239	915	
—	289	893	2401		—	—	562	421	
—	(8.6)	(11.9)	(10.4)		—	—	(13.3)	(13.2)	
4.7	18.8	—	20.0	0.144	4.5	12.5	—	32.6	
—	11.4	32.4	13.0		—	—	32.0	—	
—	—	23.9	—		—	—	—	—	
—	—	15.2	—		—	—	—	—	
100	*1856*	*122500*	*2470*		*100*	*>100*	*≫100*	*≫100*	
—	2912	272000	4482		—	—	—	—	
—	1212	66175	1535		—	—	—	—	
—	(10.6)	(12.3)	(10.0)		—	—	—	—	

^{131}I uptake percentages probably were in the "shoulder" of the dose-response curve as the individual uptake percentages, especially with the high dose (range 28.6% to 74.2%).

and consequently of difficulties in the interpretation of the assay results. It was hoped to obtain some information on the success or failure to separate this interfering principle from the supernatants used for the comparative assays by comparing the thyroid uptakes of ^{131}I in castrated recipient mice with those in "intact" recipient mice induced by these supernatants. The first four assay series were therefore performed simultaneously with castrated and with "intact" recipient mice as "duplo assays". In the last two assay series only the high dose was used in the assay with castrated recipient mice.

The results of the "repeat" experiment and all the subsequent assays using the Sn 14,000 $\times$ g are given in Table 19. The comparative assays showed that the two treatments, which aim at a deprivation of thyroid hormone resulted in a substantial increase of the pituitary content of TSH. No significant differences in this respect were found between "radiothyroidectomy" and methylthiouracil treatment during the first six months after starting treatment. The assays, which were carried out at the time that "radiothyroidectomy" had caused tumourous enlargement of the pituitary, however, showed a pronounced difference: The TSH content of the "radiothyroidectomy" pituitaries had increased more than 1000 fold, whereas that of the "methyltiouracil pituitaries" increased only 25- to 50 fold over the TSH content of the "control" pituitaries. The effect of oestrone treatment appeared to differ in the two strains of mice used as pituitary donors. In the BC_3H_f strain oestrone did not affect the TSH content, whereas in the Bd_f strain it led to an increase of this hormone in the pituitary. In the tumourous stage a 18.5 fold increase over the "control" pituitary was found. The amount of TSH per unit weight in the tumourous "oestrone" pituitaries was comparable to that in the "control" pituitaries of Bd_f mice. During the "pre-tumourous" stage comprising the assay experiments at 9 weeks and 23 weeks after starting treatment in Bd_f mice, a 5 fold increase of the TSH content of the "oestrone" pituitaries was indicated by the assays on "intact" recipient mice, whereas the "duplo assays" on castrated recipients failed to give any evidence that oestrone treatment had effected a change in the amount of TSH in the pituitaries.

4. Discussion

The preliminary experiments indicated that crude mouse pituitary material, namely fresh pituitaries homogenated in physiological saline, was not suitable for a comparative TSH-assay. At least two interfering substances appeared to offer difficulties in the interpretation of the results and make a true approximation of the ratios of the amount of TSH in various homogenates impossible. Centrifugation of pituitary homogenates was found to be a suitable method to separate these interfering substances from TSH. Apparently in freshly prepared homogenates of normal mouse pituitaries the following conditions existed to a fair degree: a) TSH either was contained in sub-cellular structures, which are too small to be spun down by the centrifugal force used or permeated quantitatively into the physiological saline before supernatant and precipitate were separated; b) the interfering substances were contained quantitatively in sub-cellular structures that are precipitated by the centrifugal force used and do not permeate into the supernatant. Comparison of the assay results of the experiments in which unintentionally a centrifugal force of 24,000 × g had been used with the results of the subsequent experiments using a smaller centrifugal force provided suggestive evidence that the treatments to which the donor mice had been subjected affected these conditions. For instance all assays of 14,000 × g supernatants of "methylthiouracil-" and of "radiothyroidectomy"-homogenates comprising 12 assays on "intact" and 12 assays on castrated recipient mice indicated that both treatments resulted in a substantial increase of the TSH content of the pituitary. Compared with these unequivocal results the assays using the 24,000 × g yielded inconsistent information. This suggested that the use of the larger centrifugal force had caused a nearly complete loss of TSH by spinning down the "coarser" TSH-containing particles in the "radiothyroidectomy pituitary" homogenates of the first and third assay series and from the "methylthiouracil pituitary" homogenates of the second and third series (Table 18). The extremely strong potency of the 24,000 × g supernatant of the "methylthiouracil pituitary" homogenate of the first assay series and the strong TSH potency of that of the "radiothyroidectomy pituitary" homogenate of the second series might be interpreted to reflect a diffusion of the greater part of the hormone occurring before the separation of the supernatant from the precipitated particles.

The possibility that even after centrifuging the homogenates at 14,000 × g a partial loss of TSH had occurred could not be excluded. The other cause of "negative error" inherent to the method of centrifugation is the failure to obtain a sufficient separation of the interfering substances. In the majority of "duplo assays" using the 14,000 × g supernatants the thyroid uptakes of ^{131}I in the "intact" recipient mice either did not differ from, or even were significantly higher than in the castrated recipient mice. This suggested that the separation of the second interfering principle (V. A. 3. d.) had been only partially achieved. Especially in the case of homogenates of pituitaries of oestrone-treated Bd_f mice this resulted in a considerable difference in the estimates of their TSH contents between the assays using castrated recipient mice and the "duplo assays" using "intact" recipient mice.

The method of centrifugation of pituitary homogenates therefore appeared not suitable for a *true* approximation of the ratios of the TSH contents of pituitaries of variously treated mice. The use of the supernatant for the comparative assay experiments, however, may be considered a real improvement over the use of crude pituitary material, e.g. "total homogenate", etc. In the early stage of the development of the assay method "total homogenate" of pituitary tumours induced by "radiothyroidectomy" had been compared with that of "control" pituitaries in this institute (unpublished experiments, J. Moeljono, 1953). The results of these early experiments had been equivocal; the thyroid uptakes of ^{131}I induced by "radiothyroidectomy tumour" homogenate had been the same or only slightly higher than that induced by the "control pituitary" homogenate. In one assay only a significantly higher uptake had been induced by the tumour homogenate. In this particular experiment the rather massive dose of the equivalent of 12 mg of pituitary tumour (wet weight) per injection had been compared with the equivalent of 0.2 mg of a normal pituitary per injection. The ^{131}I uptakes by the thyroids had been 25.7% and 10.1% respectively. In the present experiments the lowest dose of "radiothyroidectomy tumour" homogenate injected was the equivalent of 1/1,500 of a pituitary tumour, which was approximately 0.02 mg of pituitary tumour tissue (wet weight), per injection. This low dose resulted in a thyroid uptake of ^{131}I of 15.2% in recipient mice that received cortisone simultaneously. Since cortisone "flattens" the slope of the dose-response curve and cortisone had not been used in the early experiments, the difference between the early and the present experiments is even more remarkable. It appears justifiable to attribute the difference in "TSH potency" of the "pituitary tumour" homogenates found between the early and the present experiments to the use of the 14,000 × g supernatant and the separation of interfering substances that was obtained by centrifuging the homogenate. Supportive evidence for an extremely high TSH content of "radiothyroidectomy"-induced pituitary tumours came from the PAS reaction (see IV. B. 2.). The results with the modified PAS technique on pituitary tumour sections were consistent with the estimate of a 40- to 100 fold increase of the amount of TSH per unit weight in tumour tissue in respect to normal pituitary tissue.

In Table 20 a comparison has been made between the estimates of the TSH content of "radiothyroidectomy"-induced pituitary tumours by BATES, ANDERSON and FURTH (1957) and the present experiments.

Table 20. *TSH assay of primary "radiothyroidectomy"-induced pituitary tumours in mice*

	BATES and co-workers	Present experiments
Strain of mice used	C_{57}Bl	(C_{57}Bl × C_3H_f) F_1 (C_{57}Bl × DBA_f) F_1
time after "radio-thyroidectomy"	1 year	53 weeks 46 weeks
weight range of pituitary tumours	20—90 mg	20—60 mg 16—45 mg
estimated ratio of TSH content per unit weight of pit. tum. : norm. pit.	1 : 1	> 40 : 1
estimated TSH content of normal mouse pituitary	0.04—0.08 USP	(C_{75}Bl × C_3H_f) F_1 : ± 0.02 (C_{75}Bl × DBA_f) F_1 : ± 0.03 (WLL_f × O_{20}) F_1 : ± 0.07
assay method:		
1. assay animal	day-old chick (not the same species as the pituitary donor animal)	hypophysectomized mice (same species, or even same species and same strain)
2. parameter of thyroid stimulation	^{131}I depletion	^{131}I uptake

The American experiments showed somewhat higher estimates of the TSH content of normal mouse pituitaries. In this respect it is interesting that PAS-positive cells have been stated (HALMI and GUDE, 1954) to make up less than 10% of the cell population of the normal mouse pituitary (C_{57}Bl), whereas even with the very sensitive PAS modification used in the present material less than 1% of the cell population of the normal mouse pituitary showed PAS-positive granules. The difference between the amounts of TSH found in the normal pituitary, however, is far too small to account for the salient difference in the estimate of the amount of TSH per unit weight of tumourous tissue in respect to normal pituitary tissue. The limitations of the chick assay for biological material has been reported (POSTEL, 1956; GREENSPAN and LEW, 1959). Of special interest is the demonstration of fractions, which inhibit the end point of this bioassay, in crude pituitary material by POSTEL.

The correlation of the results of the present assay for TSH and the amount of glycoprotein granules disclosed by the modification of the PAS staining was almost conclusive evidence that the TSH content per unit-weight in primary ^{131}I induced pituitary tumours had increased tremendously. The inference was that the principles, which have been presumed to be present in normal mouse pituitaries and which modulate the effect of TSH on ^{131}I uptake of the thyroid gland, were present in the tumourous pituitaries in sufficient amounts to mask the increase in TSH. It justified a discussion of their possible mode of action.

The first principle (see V. A. 3. b.) inhibited thyroid uptake of ^{131}I in recipient mice of the Od_f strain and enhanced it in those of the Bd_f strain. These opposite modulating effects on ^{131}I uptake could be imitated by administering small doses of ACTH (8 γ) to mice of these two strains concurrently with TSH injections. More massive doses of ACTH (70 γ) had an inhibitive effect in both strains of mice. Since cortisone (10 γ) inhibited ^{131}I uptake induced by TSH in both strains of mice, the inhibition of ^{131}I uptake by ACTH might be attributable to induction of endogenous cortisone production. The mechanism by which the smaller dose of ACTH enhanced ^{131}I uptake in hypophysectomized mice of the Bd_f strain remained a matter of conjecture. There was no indication that the comparative TSH-assays using the 14,000 $\times$ g supernatants had been interfered by this "ACTH like" principle. No appreciable differences in the slopes of the dose-response curves were found, whereas this "ACTH like" principle might be expected to flatten the slope appreciably if it acts via endogenous cortisone production.

The second principle (see V. A. 3. d.) inhibited thyroid uptake of ^{131}I induced by TSH in castrated recipient mice particularly. Prolactin administered concurrently with TSH was shown to inhibit ^{131}I uptake induced by TSH significantly in castrated recipient mice in doses that did not appear to affect ^{131}I uptake in "intact" recipients. Comparison of ^{131}I uptakes in castrated and "intact" recipient mice suggested that this second, "prolactin like", principle had only been partially separated from the supernatants of most of the "experimental" homogenates by the centrifugal force used. This was most distinct in the pituitary homogenates of oestrone-treated Bd_f mice. These "oestrone" supernatants induced significantly higher ^{131}I uptakes in the "intact" recipient mice than in the castrated ones, suggesting that they contained sufficient amounts of this "prolactin like" principle to interfere with the TSH-assay. Since it is generally accepted that the pituitary under oestrone stimulation elaborates predominantly prolactin (WOLFE, BRYAN and WRIGHT, 1938; LACOUR, 1959; MÜHLBOCK, 1953; MEYER and CLIFTON, 1956), this provided supportive evidence for the inference that the second principle is closely linked to prolactin or might be prolactin itself. It seems probable that this "prolactin like" principle is the major cause of false, too low, estimates of TSH. The assay results with the Bd_f "oestrone" supernatants demonstrated that an increase in pituitary TSH can be masked to a considerable extent. The TSH ratio between "oestrone" and "control" supernatants calculated from the ^{131}I uptakes in "intact" recipient mice should be considered to give the best approximation, because the uptakes in the "intact" recipient mice are not affected, or less affected, by a contamination of the assay material with this principle. Oestrone treatment of Bd_f mice resulted (9 weeks and 23 weeks after starting treatment) in an increase of pituitary TSH, which should be estimated to be at least 2.8[1] times the amount of TSH in the normal pituitary. This increase was totally masked, presumably by the contamination with the "prolactin like" principle in the supernatant containing TSH, in the "duplo assay" using castrated recipients. It suggested that oestrone administration resulted in an increase in prolactin, which may be accompanied by a less distinct increase in TSH. The observations on the ^{131}I uptakes induced in "intact" and in castrated recipients by the "radiothyroidectomy"- and the "methylthiouracil-supernatants" suggested that a deficiency of thyroid hormone caused an increase in TSH that probably is accompanied by an increase in prolactin or a "prolactin like" substance.

Although apparently the "prolactin like" substance had been separated from the various supernatants with varying degrees of success, the slope of the assays did not differ more than could be expected from experimental variance. Contamination of the TSH in the assay material with this presumed principle therefore appeared not to affect the slope of the dose-response curve. This suggested that the inhibitive action on thyroid uptake of ^{131}I, which was caused by this principle resulted in too low estimates of TSH by effecting a parallel shift of the dose-response curve rather than by flattening the slope of the curve. This may be demonstrated by the ^{131}I uptakes obtained with the supernatants of homogenated pituitaries of "radiothyroidectomized" and of methylthiouracil-treated mice of the Bd_f strain 23 weeks after starting treatment. In these assay series the estimates of the TSH potency of the "radiothyroidectomy" supernatant of the "duplo assay" did not differ significantly, since the 5% fiducial limits overlap. The estimates of the TSH potency of the "methylhiouracil" supernatant, however, differed approximately by a factor 8. This difference cannot be accounted for by experi-

[1] The lower of the 5% fiducial limits (see table 19).

mental variance, since the 5% fiducial limits, being 12,000% to 2,401% and 915% to 421% in the assay on "intact" and on castrated recipients respectively, do not overlap. Comparison of the thyroid uptakes of ^{131}I induced by these two supernatants in the "intact" and the castrated recipient mice suggested that the "methylthiouracil" supernatant was contaminated with the "prolactin like" principle, whereas the "radiothyroidectomy" supernatant apparently was free.

If it is presumed that the assay using "intact" recipients is correct, the TSH ratio for 1/60 "radiothyroidectomy"-; 1/60 "methylthiouracil"-;

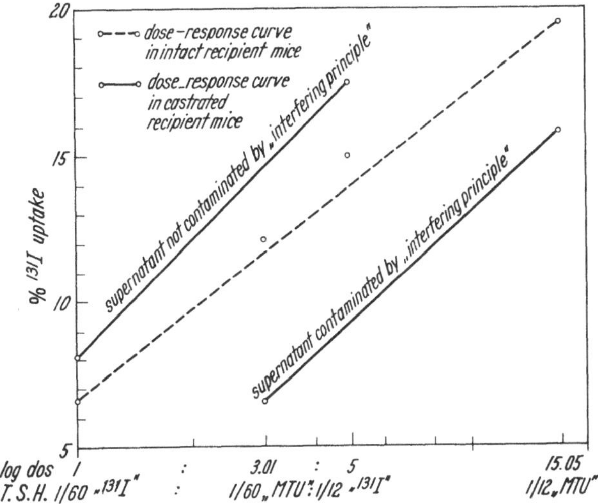

Fig. 16. „Shift" of dose-response curve in castrated recipient mice

1/12 "radiothyroidectomy"- and 1/12 "methylthiouracil"-doses can be calculated to be 1 : 3 : 5 : 15. When the logarithms of the calculated TSH ratios are then plotted against the percentage of administered ^{131}I, which the doses of these two supernatants induced to be taken up by the thyroids of the castrated recipients, two parallel lines will result. The parallel shift thus demonstrated (Fig. 16) must be attributed to the "prolactin like" principle in the "methylthiouracil" supernatant. This would be consistent with a "competetive inhibition" between the "prolactin-like" principle and TSH suggesting a common molecular configuration between them. Such a common molecular configuration between TSH and "prolactin" theoretically may have the following two bearings upon pituitary patho-physiology: a) It suggest a mechanism by which a serious disturbance in one of the various systems of interplay between the pituitary and its target gland (e.g. between pituitary and gonads) may upset the negative feed-back mechanism in another of these systems of interplay (e.g. between pituitary and thyroid) (see Fig. 17). b) Together with the findings discussed in the preceeding two chapters, the following concept of the pituitary gland appears possible: Pituitary cells on which the hypothalamus does not exert a differentiational effect, produce the "mother hormone". This "mother hormone", from experiments quoted in the above mentioned chapters, appears to have a predominantly prolactin like action. Under the influence of stimuli from the hypothalamus enzyme systems in these pituitary cells may become activated and break off parts of the "mother hormone" that have TSH-, FSH-, LH-, ACTH-,

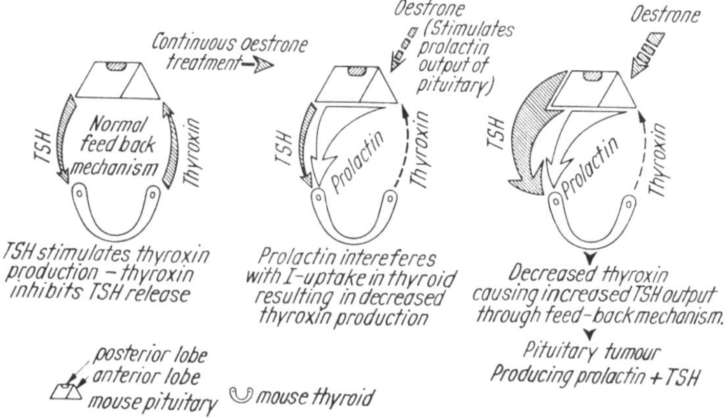

Fig. 17. Postulated mechanism of enhanced TSH-production by continuous oestrone administration in the Bdf F_1 strain

or STH (growth hormone)-like activities respectively. Thus the monocellular concept of the pituitary gland may be brought in agreement with modern concepts of the hypothalamo-pituitary relationship.

5. Summary

Preliminary experiments indicated the presence in crude pituitary material of substances that can modify the effect of TSH on the ^{131}I uptake in the thyroids of hypophysectomized mice. Centrifugation of normal pituitaries homogenated in physiological saline can separate these substances from the supernatant fraction containing TSH. Centrifugation appeared to be unreliable in this respect, however, if the pituitaries came from treated mice. A true approximation of the TSH ratios between normal pituitaries and pituitaries obtained from "radiothyroidectomized"-, methylthiouracil-treated and oestrone-treated mice therefore probably was not attained. The separation of interfering substances by centrifugation, although not complete, appeared to have resulted in a real improvement over the use of crude pituitary material for comparative TSH-assays: for example results with the modified PAS technique on sections of pituitary tumours induced by "radiothyroidectomy" supported the finding of enormous increases of TSH (more than 1000 fold) disclosed by the assays using the supernatant fraction of such tumours. As long as the pituitary glands of methylthiouracil-treated and "radiothyroidectomized mice did not differ significantly in weight, the increase in pituitary TSH was found to be approximately of the same magnitude, ranging from 4- to 40 fold, irrespective of the treatment causing the thyroid hormone deficiency. In assays using crude pituitary material apparently this increase was masked to a great extent.

Oestrone treatment was found to increase pituitary TSH content in one strain and did not affect it in the other strain of mice used as pituitary donor mice. The assay experiments are considered to indicate that in mice of the first strain the hormonal imbalance in the gonadal-pituitary feed-back system leading to an excessive prolactin output upsets the thyroid-pituitary interrelation by a "competitive inhibition" by the excess of prolactin interfering with the action of TSH on the thyroid gland.

VI. General Summary

An outline is given of the recent trend to conceive normal growth and normal cell replacement as a balance between the "organizing forces" of the organism and the "inherent growth potentialities" of its various types of cells. In such a view cancerous growth therefore is a failure of these "organizing forces" to keep the "inherent" (or as an alternative possibility: the newly acquired) growth potentialities of a cell (or a group of cells) in check and tuned to the demand of the organism. This concept appeared to be especially suitable for the study of pituitary tumours.

The literature pertaining to pituitary tumours, spontaneous and induced, in mice and rats is reviewed. The genetical constitution appears to influence the incidence and a "hormonal imbalance" is thought to have been operative in the development of spontaneous pituitary tumours and also appears to be the distinctive feature common to most procedures that are followed by development of pituitary tumours. Two extreme views are discussed, namely a) that pituitary tumours are derived from functionnally and morphologically irreversibly differentiated, monohormonal cells and b) that such tumours consist of "hormonally multipotent" cells. A survey of the data showed that a constant relationship between a well established type of "hormonal imbalance" and a definite functional type of pituitary tumour is restricted to that between hyperoestrogenization and tumours producing prolactin on the one hand and that between thyroid hormone deprivation and tumours producing TSH on the other hand. A comparative study of the various characteristics of the two mentioned types of pituitary tumours appeared to be a useful approach to an assesment of the conflicting views about the nature and origin of pituitary tumours in general.

The influence on incidence and on growth rate of experimental pituitary tumours of the genetical constitution on the one hand and of the type of "hormonal imbalance" on the other hand was studied. It was found that in one of the highly inbred strains studied "radiothyroidectomy" readily induces pituitary tumours and hyperoestrogenization fails to do so, whereas in the strain of rats studied hyperoestrogenization readily yielded pituitary tumours, but attempts to obtain pituitary tumours by "radiothyroidectomy" failed to give evidence of a positive correlation between treatment and pituitary tumour incidence.

Although in this particular inbred strain of mice and in the rats studied there was a clearcut divergence between the effects of hyperoestrogenization and "radiothyroidectomy", in all other strains of mice investigated the results suggested a close parallelism between the effects of the two types of "hormonal imbalance" on pituitary tumour incidence and rate of growth.

This "close parallelism" was further investigated by plotting the logarithms of the weights of the pituitaries against time. These semilogarithmically plotted "growth curves" of pituitary tumours in the various strains were then compared between oestrone induced- and "radiothyroidectomy"-induced pituitary tumours in the same strain and sex of mice on the one hand and between the various strains (and between the sexes) of mice within each treatment group on the other hand.

Whereas such growth curves differed in angle between various strains of mice (and in some strains even between the two sexes), apparently the method inducing tumourous enlargement of the pituitary did neither influence the angle of the growth curve (presumed to reflect the mitotic rate), nor the position of the "straight part of the growth curve" (presumed to reflect the percentage number of cells of the normal pituitary involved in the proliferation). Submitting the data to the analysis of co-variance emphasized this impression as there were no indications whatsoever to conclude that the "oestrone growth curve" and the "radiothyroidectomy growth curve" were not identical in each pair of comparable groups of mice.

It suggested 1. that a) the type of hormonal derangement does not influence the rate of growth of pituitary tumours, whereas b) the sex of the animal may do so, as well as c) the genetical constitution; 2. that pituitary tumour formation is an "all-or-none" phenomenon and not a graded response to an appropiate stimulus: The hypothalamus is considered to be the probable locus for the trigger mechanism of this "all-or-none" reaction; 3. that the percentage of cells of the normal pituitary that are induced to proliferate by "radiothyroidectomy" is about the same as that by hyperoestrogenization and this percentage may be estimated to be between 10% and 50% of the cell population of the normal pituitary: It therefore precludes the concept of "radiothyroidectomy"-induced tumours being exclusively derived from the TSH producing, PAS-positive, basophile cell type of the pituitary.

The morphology and the TSH content of the two types of pituitary tumours was then studied comparatively.

A comparative microscopical examination of a material consisting of 176 pituitary tumours and including both types, stained by the Mallory tri-chrome technique failed to give conclusive evidence. The results of the TSH-assays of pituitary tumours suggested that the amount of this glycoprotein hormone in the cells of the tumours induced by "radiothyroidectomy" should be sufficient to give a positive reaction with the PAS straining, provided that the sensitivity of the reaction could be improved. The modification described by RUYTER (1958) of the PAS reaction gave excellent results: The majority of cells in such tumours showed intra-cellular, PAS-positive granules, whereas the oestrone-induced pituitary tumours showed no cells containing material that stained with this sensitive PAS modification. Thus the results of this histo-chemical technique reinforced the conclusion drawn from the hormone-assay, e.g. that the content of a "radiothyroidectomy"-induced pituitary tumour (of approximately 30 mg) increased in the order of a thousandfold, or even more, compared to the TSH content of a normal mouse pituitary.

The apparent disagreement between the finding of identical "growth curves" on the one hand and the definite distinction between the two types of tumours, which the TSH-assays and the histo-chemical approach showed on the other hand, suggested that: 1. pituitary tumours result from cutting out the inhibitive influence of the hypothalamus on the mitotic rate of pituitary cells; 2. the hormonal function of such pituitary tumours is determined by the hormonal status of the animal bearing the tumour. (It can be assumed, however, that this will be dependent on the unimpaired functional status of the various hypothalamic centres that regulate the different pituitary functions. Pressure damage of these centres may be the cause that the cells of very large (100 mg or more) pituitary tumours induced by "radiothyroidectomy either do not show the PAS reaction any more or only show a weakly positive PAS reaction in a few scattered cells.)

On the cellular level it suggested that either a) a reasonably large percentage of undifferentiated cells exists along with the fully differentiated ones in the normal mouse pituitary and that these are the cells that give rise to the pituitary tumours and differentiate according to the prevailing hormonal status of the tumour bearing animal; or that b) the differentiation into functionally and morphologically different types of cells, such as the prolactin-producing-eosinophile cell or the TSH-producing-basophile cell, is not an irreversible one.

Although the various experiments described in chapters III, IV and V do not necessarily preclude the concept of the various types of pituitary tnmours originating from the functionally corresponding cell type in the nurmal pituitary. They provided, however, suggestive evidence in favour of a concept that each of them may originate from more than one cell type, or that they originate from a hormonally multipotent cell type. The TSH-assay experiments, which indicated an interfering action between various pituitary hormones and TSH suggested that at least between "prolactin" and TSH it was probably due to some "common specific molecular configuration" in their peptide chains. This would fit into the following view on the sub-cellular level: Pituitary cells produce a "mother substance" or "mother hormone" when the hypothalamus does not exert its differentiational effects. Stimuli from the hypothalamic centres activate enzyme systems in the pituitary cells and the "mother hormone" is then further processed and the cell secretes substances that have TSH-, FSH-, LH-, ACTH- or STH (growth hormone)-like activities respectively as the case may be.

The outline of the above "monocellular" concept of the origin of pituitary tumours is not given as an established theory, but rather as a working hypothesis that has emerged from the experiences described in the present work and that may serve as a starting point for further experiments envisaged in the Netherland's Cancer Institute.

As to the nature of the pituitary tumours, it appears that to many the following questions are of great importance: whether it is a hyperplastic or a neoplastic process; if a neoplastic one, when the qualitative change has taken place. It has been empasized that in the view (outlined in the first chapter) of the relationship between normal growth and cell replacement on the one hand and neoplasia on the other hand, such questions become relatively less important. The heated discussions, which these questions so often have provoked can be attributed to different definitions of terminology used by pathologists clinicians and experimental workers, etc. The virtual absence of an "apparent stationnary period" indicated by the present experiments will suggest to many that the process is of a hyperplastic nature, because it means that the proliferative process induced by the "hormonal imbalances" involves many cells at once. HERTZ (1957) has drawn attention to the fact that hyperplastic growth induced by hormones is a graded response[1], whereas hormone-induced neoplastic growth always appears to be an "all-or-none" phenomenon. Arguments have been put forward that pituitary tumour growth also is such an "all-or-none" phenomenon. Evidently pituitary tumours are in the borderland between "normal" hyperplasia and neoplasia and it therefore depends on one's definitions of these terms, whether these tumours be considered as neoplastic.

References

ADAMS, A. E.: Quart. Rev. Biol. **21**, 1 (1946).
D'ANGELO, S. A.: Endocrinology **52**, 331 (1953).
— Brookhaven Symposia **7**, 9 (1954).
— A. S. GORDON and H. A. CHARIPPER: Endocrinology **31**, 217 (1942).
ARON, M., VAN C. CAULAERT, and J. STAHL: C. R. Soc. Biol. (Paris) **107**, 64 (1931).
AXELRAD, A. A., and C. P. LEBLOND: Cancer **8**, 339 (1955).
BARRNETT, R. J., A. J. LADMAN, N. J. MCALLASTER and E. R. SIPERSTEIN: Endocrinology **59**, 398 (1956).
BATES, R. W., E. ANDERSON and J. FURTH: Endocrinology **61**, 549 (1957).
— K. H. CLIFTON and E. ANDERSON: Proc. Soc. exp. Biol. (N. Y.) **93**, 525 (1956).
BIELSCHOWSKY, F.: Brit. J. exp. Path. **25**, 90 (1944).
— Brit. J. Cancer (London) **7**, 203 (1953).
— Brit. J. Cancer (London) **8**, 154 (1954).
BIELSCHOWSKY, M., F. BIELSCHOWSKY and D. LINDSAY: Brit. J. Cancer (London) **10**, 688 (1956).
BISKIND, M. S., and G. S. BISKIND: Proc. Soc. exp. Biol. (N. Y.) **55**, 176 (1944).
BOGDANOVE, E. M., and S. A. D'ANGELO: Endocrinology **64**, 123 (1959).
BOOT, L. M., and O. MÜHLBOCK: Acta Un. int. Cancr. **12**, 577 (1956).
— — Acta Un. int. Cancr. **15**, 134 (1959).
BROWN, J. H., and M. HESS: Amer. J. Physiol. **188**, 25 (1957).
BROWN, R. W., D. M. WOODBURY and G. SAYERS: J. clin. Endocr. **12**, 939 (1952).
BROWN-GRANT, K.: CIBA-foundation colloquia on Endocrinol. **10**, 97 (1957).
BRYAN, W. R., G. H. KLINCK and J. M. WOLFE: Amer. J. Cancer **33**, 370 (1938).

[1] The hyperplastic growth induced in target glands by hormones in fact is such a well graded response that it has served in several instances as the bases of a quantitative hormone assay (e.g. the ventral prostate of hypophysectomized rats for LH-assay).

BURT, A. S., B. H. LANDING and S. C. SOMMERS: Cancer Res. **14**, 497 (1954).
CALAPA, F.: Minerva ginec. (Torino) **2**, 521 (1950).
CASAS, C. B., and E. KOPPISCH: Endocrinology **51**, 322 (1952).
CHAMORRO, A.: Ann. Endocr. (Paris) **8**, 330 (1947).
CH'EN, G., and H. B. VAN DYKE: Chin. J. Physiol. **10**, 285 (1936).
CLAUSEN, H. J.: Growth **20**, 213 (1956).
CLIFTON, K. H.: Cancer Res. **19**, 2 (1959).
— and J. FURTH: Fed. Proc. **15**, 512 (1956).
— and R. K. MEYER: Endocrinology **58**, 681 (1956a).
— — Anat. Rec. **125**, 65 (1956b).
COLLIP, J. B.: quoted in: The Physiological Basis of Medical Practice, p. 784, footnote. Baltimore: C. H. Best & N. B. Taylor; the Williams and Wilkins Cy., 1955.
COWIE, A. T., and S. J. FOLLEY: in: The Hormones, vol. III pp. 309—379. New York: Eds. G. Pincus & K. V. Thimann; Acad. Press Inc. Publ., 1955.
CRAMER, W., and E. S. HORNING: Lancet **230**, 247 (1936a).
— — Lancet **230**, 1056 (1936b).
— — Lancet **234**, 72 (1938).
CROWE, S. J., H. CUSHING and J. HOMANS: Bull. Johns Hopk. Hosp. **21**, 127 (1910).
CURTIS, M. R., F. D. BULLOCK and H. S. DUNNING: Amer. J. Cancer **26**, 67 (1936).
DALTON, A. J., H. P. MORRIS and C. S. DUBNIK: J. nat. Cancer Inst. **9**, 201 (1949).
DAWSON, A. B.: Amer. J. Anat. **78**, 347 (1946).
DEL CONTE, E., and M. STUX: Acta endocr. (Copenhagen) **20**, 246 (1955).
DENT, J. N., E. L. GADSDEN and J. FURTH: Cancer Res. **15**, 70 (1955).
— — — Cancer Res. **16**, 171 (1956).
DESCLIN, L.: C. R. Soc. Biol. (Paris) **146**, 781 (1952).
— and A. M. ERMANS: C. R. Soc. Biol. (Paris) **144**, 1277 (1950).
DICKIE, M. M., and P. W. LANE: Cancer Res. **16**, 48 (1956).
— and G. W. WOOLLEY: Cancer Res. **9**, 372 (1949).
DIXON, W. J., and F. J. MASSEY: Introduction to Statistical Analysis. New York: McGraw-Hill 1957.
DYKE, D. C. VAN, M. E. SIMPSON, A. A. KONEFF and C. A. TOBIAS: Endocrinology **64**, 240 (1959).
EBBENHORST-TENGBERGEN, W. J. P. R. VAN: Acta endocr. (Copenhagen) **18**, 213 (1955).
ECK, W. F. VAN: Thesis. Amsterdam 1940.
EDELMANN, A.: Brookhaven Symposium in Biology **7**, 250 (1955).
EEDEN, C. VAN: Statistica ('s Gravenhage) **7**, 141 (1953).
— and CHR. L. RÜMKE: Statistica Neerlandica **12**, 265 (1958).
ENGEL, F. L.: Yale J. Biol. Med. **30**, 201 (1957).
EPSTEIN, D., A. CANTAROW, G. FRIEDLER, and K. E. PASCHKIS: Proc. Soc. exp. Biol. (N. Y.) **82**, 50 (1953).
— and L. F. WOLTERINK: Poultry Science **28**, 763 (1949).
EVANS, H. M., and M. E. SIMPSON: Amer. J. Physiol. **89**, 371 (1929).
EVERETT, J. W.: Endocrinology **58**, 786 (1956).
FIELD, E. J.: J. Anat. (Lond.) **92**, 137 (1958).
FREUDENBERGER, C. B., and F. W. CLAUSEN: Anat. Rec. **69**, 171 (1937).
FRY, E. G., M. MILLER and C. N. H. LONG: Endocrinology **30**, 1029 (1942).
FURTH, J.: Cancer Res. **13**, 477 (1953).
— Amer. J. Path. **30**, 421 (1954a).
— J. nat. Cancer Inst. **15**, 687 (1954b).
— Recent Progress in Hormone Research, New York, Academie Press: ed. G. Pincus **11**, 221 (1955).
— Cancer Res. **17**, 454 (1957).
— R. F. BUFFETT and E. L. GADSDEN: Proc. Amer. Ass. Cancer Res. **2**, 204 (1957).
— — and N. HARAN-GHERA: Acta Un. int. Cancr. **16**, 138 (1960).
— and W. T. BURNETT: Proc. Soc. exp. Biol. (N. Y.) **78**, 222 (1951).
— — and E. L. GADSDEN: Cancer Res. **13**, 298 (1953).
— and K. H. CLIFTON: CIBA-foundation colloquia on Endocrinology **12**, 3 (1958).
— — E. L. GADSDEN and R. F. BUFFETT: Cancer Res. **16**, 608 (1956).
— J. N. DENT, W. T. BURNETT and E. L. GADSDEN: J. clin. Endocr. **15**, 81 (1955).

FURTH, J., E. L. GADSDEN and W. T. BURNETT: Proc. Soc. exp. Biol. (N. Y.) **80**, 4, (1952).
— — Fed. Proc. **14**, 403 (1955).
— — K. H. CLIFTON and E. ANDERSON: Cancer Res. **16**, 600 (1956).
— — and A. C. UPTON: Proc. Soc. exp. Biol. (N. Y.) **84**, 253 (1953).
GABRILOVE, J. L., W. R. DORRANCE and L. J. SOFFER: Amer. J. Physiol. **169**, 565 (1952).
GADDUM, J. H.: Pharmacol. Rev. **5**, 87 (1953).
GADSDEN, E. L., and J. FURTH: Proc. Soc. exp. Biol. (N. Y.) **83**, 511 (1953).
GARDNER, W. U.: Cancer Res. **1**, 345 (1941).
— Cancer Res. **8**, 397 (1948a).
— Acta Un. int. Cancr. **6**, 124 (1948b).
— Advanc. Cancer Res. **1**, 173 (1953).
— C. A. PFEIFFER, J. J. TRENTIN and J. T. WOLSTENHOLME: The Physiopathology of Cancer p. 225 New-York: eds. F. Homburger & W. H. Fishman; Hoeber-Harper Inc. 1953.
— G. M. SMITH and L. C. STRONG: Amer. J. Cancer **26**, 541 (1936).
GILLMAN, J., and CH. GILBERT: Nature (London) **175**, 724 (1955).
GOLDBERG, R. C., and I. L. CHAIKOFF: Endocrinology **48**, 1 (1951).
— — Anat. Rec. **112**, 265 (1952).
GORBMAN, A.: Cancer Res. **7**, 746 (1947).
— Proc. Soc. exp. Biol. (N. Y.) **71**, 237 (1949).
— J. clin. Endocr. **10**, 1177 (1950).
— Proc. Soc. exp. Biol. (N. Y.) **80**, 538 (1952).
— Cancer Res. **16**, 99 (1956).
— and A. EDELMANN: Proc. Soc. exp. Biol. (N. Y.) **81**, 348 (1952).
GORDON, A. S., E. D. GOLDSMITH and H. A. CHARIPPER: Endocrinology **36**, 53 (1945).
GREENSPAN, F. S., and W. LEW: Endocrinology **64**, 160 (1959).
GRIESBACH, W. E., and H. D. PURVES: Brit. J. exp. Path. **24**, 174 (1943).
— — Brit. J. exp. Path. **26**, 13 (1945).
HALMI, N. S.: Endocrinology **47**, 4 (1950).
— Endocrinology **50**, 1 (1952a).
— Anat. Rec. **112**, 1 (1952b).
— and W. D. GUDE: Amer. J. Path. **30**, 403 (1954).
HARRIS, G. W.: Neutral Control of the Pituitary Gland. London: Arnold 1955.
HARRIS, J. I., and A. B. LEARNER: Nature (London) **179**, 1346 (1957).
HERLANT, M.: Ann. Endocr. (Paris) **13**, 611 (1952).
HERTZ, R.: Cancer Res. **17**, 423 (1957).
HOHLWEG, W., and K. JUNKMANN: Pflügers Arch. ges. Physiol. **232**, 148 (1933).
HORNING, E. S.: Oestrogens and Neoplasia, p. 43. Oxford: eds. H. Burrows & E. S. Horning, Blackwell Scientific Publications 1952.
HOSKINS, R. G.: J. clin. Endocr. **9**, 1429 (1949).
HOUSSAY, B. A.: C. R. Soc. Biol. (Paris) **111**, 459 (1932).
— A. B. HOUSSAY, A. F. CARDEZA and R. M. PINTO: Schweiz. med. Wschr. **85**, 291 (1955).
— A. NOVELLI and R. SAMMARTINO: C. R. Soc. Biol. (Paris) **111**, 830 (1932).
KAPLAN, H. S.: Acta Un. int. Cancr. **15**, 543 (1959a).
— Cancer Res. **19**, 791 (1959b).
KIEF, H.: Beitr. path. Anat. **116**, 541 (1956).
KONEFF, A. A., D. C. VAN DYKE and H. M. EVANS: Endocrinology **51**, 249 (1952).
KUSCHINSKY, G.: Naunyn-Schmiedebergs Arch. exp. Path. Pharmak. **170**, 510 (1933).
KWA, H. G.: Acta physiol. pharmacol. neerl. 8, 1 (1959).
LACOUR, F.: C. R. Soc. Biol. (Paris) **144**, 248 (1950).
LADMAN, A. J., and R. J. BARRNETT: Endocrinology **54**, 355 (1954).
— — J. Morph. **98**, 305 (1956).
LAMEYER, L. D. F.: Thesis. Leiden 1956.
LAQUEUR, E., P. C. HART and S. E. DE JONGH: Dtsch. med. Wschr. **44**, 876 (1926).

LEBEDEWA, N. S.: Naunyn-Schmiedeberg's Arch. exp. Path. Pharmak. **183**, 15 (1936).
LEHMAN, H.: Arch. Physiol. **216**, 729 (1927).
LORAINE, J. A.: The Clinical Application of Hormone Assay, Edinburgh and London: E. & S. Livingstone Ltd. 1958.
McEUEN, C. S., H. SELYE and J. B. COLLIP: Lancet **230**, 775 (1936).
McQUILLAN, M. T., V. M. TRIKOJUS, A. D. CAMPBELL and A. W. TURNER: Brit. J. exp. Path. **29**, 93 (1948).
MEITES, J., and C. W. TURNER: Res. Bull. agric. Exp. Stat. Missouri, 415 (1948).
MELLGREN, J.: Acta path. microbiol. scand. (suppl. 60) **22**, 1 (1945).
MERCIER-PAROT, L., and H. TUCHMANN-DUPLEISIS: C. R. Soc. Biol. (Paris) **148**, 449 (1954).
MEYER, R. K., and K. H. CLIFTON: Endocrinology **58**, 686 (1956).
MONEY, W. L., L. KIRSCHNER, L. KRAINTZ, P. MERRIL and R. W. RAWSON: J. clin. Endocr. **10**, 1282 (1950).
— L. KRAINTZ, J. FAGER, L. KIRSCHNER and R. W. RAWSON: Endocrinology **48**, 682 (1951).
MOORE, C. R., and D. PRICE: Amer. J. Anat. **50**, 13 (1932).
MOORE, G. E., E. L. BRACKNEY and F. G. BOCK: Proc. Soc. exp. Biol. (N. Y.) **82**, 643 (1953).
MORRIS, H. P., C. D. GREEN and A. J. DALTON: J. nat. Cancer Inst. **11**, 805 (1951).
— L. S. LOMBARD, B. P. WAGNER and J. H. WEISBURGER: Cancer Res. **2**, 234 (1957).
MÜHLBOCK, O.: Ned. T. Geneesk. **95**, 758 (1951).
— Nederl. Kanker Jaarb. **3**, 14 (1953).
— Acta Un. int. Cancr. **15**, 1 (1959).
— and L. M. BOOT: CIBA-foundation symposium on carcinogenesis. Mechanisms of action p. 83 (1959).
— — Cancer Res. **19**, 402 (1959).
NADEL, E., E. S. JOSEPHSON and A. S. MUNLAY: Endocrinology **46**, 253 (1950).
NOACH, E. L.: Acta endocr. (Copenhagen) **19**, 127 (1955).
NOVELLI, E.: Arch. E. Maragliano pat. Clin. **7**, 273 (1952).
OBERLING, C., M. GUÉRIN and P. GUÉRIN: C. R. Soc. Biol. (Paris) **123**, 1152 (1936).
— C. SANNIE, P. GUÉRIN and M. GUÉRIN: C. R. Soc. Biol. (Paris) **131**, 455 (1939).
PASCHKIS, K. E., A. CANTAROW and W. C. PEACOCK: Proc. Soc. exp. Biol. (N. Y.) **68**, 485 (1948).
— D. EPSTEIN, A. CANTAROW and G. FRIEDLER: J. clin. Endocr. **12**, 939 (1952).
PEARSE, A. G. E.: CIBA-foundation colloquia on Endocrinology **4**, 1 (1952a).
— J. Path. Bact. **64**, 791 (1952b).
— J. Path. Bact. **64**, 811 (1952b).
— Histochemistry Theoretical and Applied, London: J. & A. Churchill 1954.
PINCUS, G. E., and N. WERTHESSEN: Amer. J. Physiol. **103**, 631 (1933).
POSTEL, SH.: Endocrinology **58**, 557 (1956).
POUMEAU-DELILLE, G.: Rev. Soc. argent. Biol. **24**, 7 (1948).
PURVES, H. D., and W. E. GRIESBACH: Endocrinology **49**, 244 (1951a).
— — Endocrinology **49**, 427 (1951b).
— — Endocrinology **56**, 374 (1955).
— — J. Endocr. **13**, 365 (1956).
— — J. Endocr. **14**, 361 (1957a).
— — CIBA-foundation colloquia on Endocrinology **10**, 51 (1957b).
QUERIDO, A., A. A. H. KASSENAAR and L. D. F. LAMEYER: Acta endocr. (Copenhagen) **12**, 335 (1953).
RENNELS, E. G., J. E. HILDEBRAND and J. C. FINERTY: Anat. Rec. **125**, 594 (1956).
RIDDLE, O.: quoted in: The Physiological Basis of Medical Practice, p. 784, footnote. Baltimore: C. H. Best & N. B. Taylor; the Williams and Wilkins Cy. 1955.
ROTHBALLER, A. B.: Neuroendocrinology, report exclusively prepared for Excerpta medica, Amsterdam: Excerpta medica, section Endocrinology 1957.
RUSSFIELD, A. B., L. REINER and H. KLAUS: Amer. J. Path. **32**, 1055 (1956).
RUYTER, J. H.: Ned. T. Geneesk. **102**, 1633 (1958a).
— Acta neerl. Morph. **2**, 110 (1958b).

SAXTON, J. A.: Cancer Res. **1**, 277 (1941).
— and J. B. GRAHAM: Cancer Res. **4**, 168 (1944).
SAYERS, G., and M. A. SAYERS: Endocrinology **40**, 265 (1947).
SEIFTER, J. W., E. EHRICH and G. M. HUDYMA: Arch. Path. (Chicago) **48**, 536 (1949).
SEVERINGHAUS, A. E.: Anat. Rec. **57**, 149 (1933).
— Physiol. Rev. **17**, 556 (1937).
SHERWOOD, T. C.: J. Nutr. **12**, 223 (1936).
SILBERBERG, R., and M. SILBERBERG: Proc. Soc. exp. Biol. (N. Y.) **85**, 448 (1954).
SLYE, M., H. F. HOLMES and H. G. WELLS: Amer. J. Cancer **15**, 1387 (1931).
SMITH, P. E.: Anat. Rec. **11**, 57 (1916).
— Anat. Rec. **32**, 221 (1926).
SMITHERS, D. W.: Lancet **1959I**, 589.
SOFFER, L. J., J. L. GABRILOVE and W. R. DORRANCE: Proc. Soc. exp. Biol. (N. Y.) **76**, 763 (1951).
STIGLIANI, R., L. MAGGI and M. FANFANI: Arch. De Vecchi Anat. pat. **22**, 821 (1954).
SYDNER, K. L., and G. SAYERS: Proc. Soc. exp. Biol. (N. Y.) **83**, 729 (1953).
TAGLIAFERRO, P.: Folia gynaec. **30**, 597 (1933).
THOMAS, F.: Endocrinology **23**, 99 (1938).
TURNER, C. W., and P. T. CUPPS: Endocrinology **26**, 1042 (1940).
UPTON, A. C., and J. FURTH: J. nat. Cancer Inst. **15**, 1005 (1955).
WAHLBERG, P.: Acta endocr. (Copenhagen) **18**, suppl. 23 (1955).
WITSCHI, E.: Symposia Quant. Biol. (Cold Spring Harbor) **5**, 180 (1937).
WOLFE, J. M.: Amer. J. Anat. **85**, 309 (1949).
— W. R. BRYAN and A. W. WRIGHT: Amer. J. Cancer **34**, 352 (1938).
ZECKWER, I. T.: Amer. J. Physiol. **117**, 518 (1936).
ZONDECK, B.: Lancet **230**, 776 (1936).